My Own Medicine

My Own Medicine

◆

The Process of Recovery from Chronic Illness

Diane Kerner

Edited by Shawn Mahshie, ClarityWorks

iUniverse, Inc.
New York Lincoln Shanghai

My Own Medicine
The Process of Recovery from Chronic Illness

iUniverse, Inc.

For information address:
iUniverse, Inc.
2021 Pine Lake Road, Suite 100
Lincoln, NE 68512
www.iuniverse.com

ISBN: 0-595-32609-9

Printed in the United States of America

To all medical providers who see beyond the bones and tendons and recognize and consider the souls of their patients.

To all the squirrels and birds, cats and dogs, trees and rivers that make it easy to feel joyful, awed, lucky and grateful in spite of the pain.

And to all my loved ones, especially Keith, whose immense love touches, inspires and gives me life—like the kiss of the fairytale prince on the lips of Sleeping Beauty. I am so blessed to be with you all in this lifetime.

Contents

Acknowledgements

I am deeply grateful to have so many mentors and angels in my life: My husband, Keith Kerner, who has been a steady, loving presence and has always believed and encouraged me to be bigger than I felt. To my amazing friends, Julie Dittmar and Ellen Jablow, for offering suggestions and helping me to get the words in the right order. And to my editor and friend of thirty years, Shawn Mahshie, for the hours and hours of conversation that inspired many of the insights in this book and whose magical tinkering made my thoughts glitter on the page.

From the medical arena, I have much gratitude that Dr. Jay Goldstein is in this world. His dedication to helping people with chronic fatigue syndrome and fibromyalgia is an incredible and generous gift. I also have a heart-full of kind words and soft feelings for Dr. Steve Clarke, who gave me the best care I have ever experienced from a medical doctor. How remarkable to find a physician who actually connects with his patients eye-to-eye and with genuine compassion, interest and openness! Dr. Clarke—I thank you every day.

Foreword

My Own Medicine speaks a truth we are ready to hear: that our epidemic of chronic conditions goes far deeper than mere diagnosis or treatment modalities; that they often *em-body* the crashing of a life that no longer fits. Such conditions require nothing short of the kind of soul-and body-driven re-invention of self Diane Kerner experienced over the course of her own multi-year battle with a curious set of debilitating symptoms and the slow rebuilding of her life.

With warmth and a subtle humor about her own process, citations and a stark level of self-honesty, Kerner details her descent into the depths of chronic fatigue syndrome, and her repeated desperate efforts to cling to the pieces of her life that had defined her thus far—eventually even clinging to the diagnosis that she ruefully realized had become her new definition of self. *My Own Medicine* details the confusion, pain, despair, acceptance, and rebuilding—in short, the experience of so many who suffer from the chronic conditions that curtail their once active lives—ending with a section that describes her own self-taught strategies for making life work.

Finally, the author unfolds her gradual—almost imperceptible, but ultimately rewarding—ascent to self-acceptance (even on the worst of days) and self-reliance on her own body and spirit for direction in healing. Courageously exploring new strategies for sustaining any progress she saw, she finally added to her list of life strategies a kind of clinging to something new—the tiny but frequent doses of joy that became her guide to a rich, full life.

Diane Kerner's new work is a refreshing must-read for sufferers of chronic conditions; who are likely to enthusiastically pass it on to their employers, friends, and family as well as the medical, mental health, and social service professionals who endeavor to help them. It will validate toward long-lost levels of self-respect, and challenge toward new levels of honesty and self-healing, all who see themselves in its truths.

This book has the power to change—on an individual and collective level—the way acquaintances and even practitioners judge, misunderstand, categorize, condescend, or cast aside those who struggle with chronic pain or illness, and to give new hope and self-trust to those who are discovering their own medicine.

Shawn Mahshie
Executive Director, ClarityWorks

Introduction

Several years after I was diagnosed with Chronic Fatigue Syndrome[1] (CFS), I began noticing changes in my illness. My remissions were lasting longer and my relapses were less severe. Some symptoms seemed to drop away and didn't show up for the relapses. Was I getting well? Was it possible to go years between relapses? My doctors couldn't say. The "experts" couldn't say. None of the books I was reading talked about much beyond symptoms, diagnosis and stabilization.

My goal in writing this book has been to bring to light the process of recovery, a much neglected aspect of the experience of CFS and many other chronic illnesses. As I write about getting well and reframing my life, it is my hope that readers will recognize some of the signposts in their own experiences and feel some uplifting of the spirit that is often devastated by the loss that comes with chronic illness.

Recovery is a process. For that reason, I have included journal entries I made throughout the more acute stages of my illness. These entries reveal that my path through CFS has not been a straight one; but rather one filled with switchbacks and dead ends. I discovered some tools along the way that helped me to slant some of the power back in my direction, and away from the virus or whatever the actual physical mechanism of CFS is. It is very physical indeed, but I learned that what you do with it mentally, emotionally and spiritually can make a huge difference.

Writing about the 'getting well' seemed less effective without describing the 'being sick.' Therefore, Section One outlines my long path to diagnosis, covering my symptoms, their impact on my life, and the many trials I encountered in the search for answers and in my multiple (futile) attempts to make the disease conform to my former way of life. It took several years for my CFS to be diagnosed,

---

1. Chronic Fatigue Syndrome (CFS) often goes by another, often preferred name, *Chronic Fatigue and Immune Dysfunction Syndrome* (CFIDS). My choice to use the abbreviated name in this book is not in any way a reflection of preference or judgment, but is simply the attraction to shortcuts that becomes such a natural reflex to those of us living with this illness. In that same spirit, my references to this illness also include Fibromyalgia, as many of us have this dual-diagnosis and the symptoms can often seem so interchangeable.

an experience many others share. Although the diagnosis was a welcome relief compared to not knowing what was wrong, I can see in retrospect some disadvantages of having been given that label. Our runaway minds begin to expect the things attached to our diagnosis and expectations have a way of becoming reality. I think it's just a part of our human nature. So I'm careful which expectations I invite to set up residence in my mind. This task requires constant vigilance and I revisit it again and again in the chapters that follow.

The second section of this book further outlines the strategies I used to adapt to my illness and to recover my happiness and sense of place in the world. Here, I break things down into five basic strategies: rest, detoxification, self-exploration, joy and finally, re-setting the mind to create an allied relationship with our thoughts and perceptions.

It is key to remember that recovery is a process of renewal and repair in which even the well among us are engaged in '24-7.' Those of us who have been hit with a long-term illness operate this principle on a more conscious level. Through my own illness I am familiar with the despair that people with CFS and other chronic illnesses experience. I understand how one's hope is diminished with each relapse of symptoms and over a long period of time with little or no measurable change for the good. I've been on the relentless pursuit of answers, as if CFS is some engineering problem that I could solve if I just had all the dimensions in front of me. I know what it's like to be frustrated by the lack of reliable information, to be swept up with the excitement of the latest treatment, to be hurt by the insensitivity or ignorance of others and to feel invalidated by all of the unknowns of CFS. I hope my story brings some of the answers closer, and that the reader is comforted by the sweet blessing of shared experience.

Did I actually get well? I consider myself mostly well now and I try not to think of myself as someone who is sick. I've applied the principles outlined in this book to the point where any limitations resulting from my illness are not readily apparent to me. I'm able to work at my job 30 hours every week, but the hours are flexible and I work many of them from home—that seems to be my threshhold if I'm going to have any other life. Instead of focusing on the fact that I can't work the usual 40-hour week, I try to notice how nice it is to have the time for other things. I was pretty darn sick for eight years and now there is this 'residue' that sometimes changes shape, but is, for the most part, predictable. As my physical discomfort decreased, I found that the cognitive symptoms of CFS—like poor memory and difficulty with concentration and complex thinking—became more prominent. My pre-illness stamina has not fully returned, but then, I have aged 15 years while ill. All in all, my life is no longer so unusual or restricted.

Being aware of this is an important point to my story. I know a lot of healthy people who 'rest' a lot more than I do! I rarely ache or run the low-grade fevers. The constantly tender and swollen glands in my neck are a thing of the past. I remain sensitive to weather changes, in particular, noticing that most of the days that I feel unwell coincide with sudden shifts from sun to rain or quick drops in the temperature. I am very tolerant of lingering symptoms; I no longer live by them. I don't stare at them. I give them less power because I don't label them as bad or permanent or let them scare me.

My therapist says that she sees CFS as a sort of adult version of "failure to thrive." It's an interesting fit with the finding that a significant number of people with CFS have backgrounds of childhood trauma. Chronic fatigue and even CFS is often listed as a symptom of Post Traumatic Stress Disorder (PTSD). People who feel helpless or hopeless in their lives for reasons other than PTSD or early childhood trauma, such as extremely sensitive persons, may also be more vulnerable than others. Because of this possible connection I think it's important for people with CFS to do some self-examination, with or without professional help, especially since resolving these conditions may result in the end of some or even all of the CFS symptoms. In the following chapters I take the reader along on my journey through some of this self-examination in the hopes that by illustrating my own very personal path, others will gain some illumination onto their own.

Those who have been ill for awhile are probably aware that no one formula or treatment has been successful at providing relief for every patient who tries it. There are many who benefit from one thing or another but no one thing that has worked for every person. Medicine so often fails to consider the vast mystery of human existence and consciousness and the influence this relatively unknown piece of the equation may have on our health and healing. I do not pretend to know what will work for others or presume that what has helped me will likewise help the reader, but I do hope that those living with chronic illness who read this book will find some strategies that bring them physical, emotional or spiritual relief.

It's hard to resist using the movie, The Wizard of Oz, as a metaphor for chronic illness, so I'll stop fighting it. Let me just say that the yellow brick road coils ahead for each of us. Whether we have CFS, fibromyalgia, multiple sclerosis, lupus or any of the others; we all seek the mighty wizard. May this book be a lantern through the darkness for all who find themselves "not in Kansas anymore."

Namaste,

—Diane

Journal Entry, June 14, 1990:

I am so tired by the variability of each day. The rare ones are sun-kissed and blessed with feelings of life and respite from despair. Most days my hope is so small and I wander into a space where walls are close and cold and there are no windows to see through to any memory of having felt better. In these times I can't imagine how I even thought—on those better days—that I might be able to add some living to my life...take a class...join a walking club...have company over for dinner.... Here I am now, chilled and achy and even the need to make a phone call feels monumentally burdensome.

And who knows me like this? No one. Because I don't answer the phone on these days or go shopping or for a visit. People see me on my good days, naturally. And who else can relate to feeling too tired to call your best friend or wash a load of towels or go out to dinner—where you're waited on—for geeminy sakes?

Section 1

The Process

One

In 1988, at thirty-five years of age, I got what I assumed was the flu. I spent the requisite three days at home and then dutifully returned to my full-time job as a special education teacher. I don't remember, but suspect, that I had used the number of days I had rested as my gauge to return to work—rather than how my body felt. I wasn't used to checking. I did what I needed to do.

When I went back to work, I noticed I still wasn't feeling too well and still had the low-grade fever and swollen glands in my neck, but figured my flu would gradually fade as it always did. Perhaps not as quickly as if I was at home in bed, but I could catch up by resting the next weekend if I had to. I could slow down the frantic pace of my life for a few more days.

Returning to work for the second week with still no improvement, even after a weekend of rest, I started getting a bit worried. I felt nagged. Why was it taking so long to get over this flu?

By this time I'd gone ahead and quit an extra, early-morning job I'd taken (teaching a sign language class before my usual full day of teaching), and had stopped the aerobic exercise I had been doing several days a week. I wasn't hanging with the after-work crowd anymore and had let the housework go a bit while I tried to rest. I saw my doctor, who ordered endless tests—repeating many of them twice, even three times. When, a couple of months later, nothing had changed, I approached my supervisor at work, Naomi, and asked for a leave so I could get more serious about rest and continue the seemingly endless doctor visits and testing that appeared to lay ahead. I had difficulty holding back my tears, felt a flood of fear as I spoke with her, and felt very grateful that my "boss" was also a good friend and someone who cared very much about me. A temporary leave would be no problem.

I was near terrified at this point. I had weird symptoms I had trouble defining and fitting into a cohesive picture; they made me fear I had something really serious. I had trouble thinking and finding words—which used to tumble out of my brain with little effort like seasoned gymnasts. Now I had to dig them out like I imagined a stroke victim would. I was always so chilled, and that could seem normal enough, but this chill came from so deep inside me and simply wouldn't resolve no matter how much time, how many blankets, or how high I set the thermostat. Rain was painful on my skin. My vision was blurred and then it wasn't. My face tingled. There were places where my skin would sting tender and raw for a couple of hours for no apparent reason and with no visible signs of irritation.

For the next three months, I went to many different doctors: internists, neurologists, psychologists, general practitioners; all were concerned at the low-grade fever I was running and the swollen, tender glands in my neck, but puzzled by the negative test results and the rather odd constellation of symptoms I presented. I slouched and hung my head in the waiting room chairs, terribly achey and barely able to stay alert.

Expensive tests showed that the pain in my wrists was caused by Carpal Tunnel Syndrome. The persistent cough was relegated to hay fever and for this I was prescribed antihistamines. My difficulty with word-finding and ordinary speech was considered a side effect of a prescription medication I had been taking for an anxiety disorder and I was taken off of it. I was being pieced out into all these independent, unrelated symptoms. It felt unsettling.

Was it possible that my entire body was falling to ruin at once, with not one explanation, but many? Could my visual, cognitive, immune, and respiratory systems all break down simultaneously yet, for unrelated reasons? I doubted that, since the onset of all of my symptoms was so sudden. Still, the doctors kept picking off one symptom at a time as if they were entirely independent of one another.

The alternating blurred vision was written off as age-related myopia, but when testing revealed that my vision was fluctuating wildly from test to test, at times *improving*, the eye doctor was certain I must be diabetic. He said that there could be no other explanation for it. But the glucose tolerance tests ruled out diabetes, as was everything else being ruled out: Rocky Mountain spotted fever, lyme disease, cat scratch fever, psittacosis, lupus, AIDS, mononucleosis, and so on. I was so weary of being poked and probed, while rather pathetically grateful for my consistent fever because it gave the doctors something tangible to observe and kept them from speculating that I was "malingering."

When I first became ill, I had been taking an antidepressant, Pamelor, for about four years to treat the depression and panic disorder that had developed some time after the death of my sister, Mary, in 1979. Mary was two years older than I was, and died from the chemotherapy that was prescribed for her leukemia, just after her twenty-ninth birthday. Her death came within months of her diagnois, as I watched and absorbed the utter fear and helplessness of the situation.

Mary had been a bit of a surrogate mother to me. When I was fourteen, my parents divorced and my mom moved out of our house. My sister took over as female head-of-household while my father was away from home much of the time, working twelve-hour shifts as a supermarket manager and sometimes dating women at night. Mary and my older brother, Joe, were protective of me, and I grew up feeling "safe" only when they were around.

By the time Mary became ill it was 1979. I was 25 years old. Mary, my older brother, Joe, and I had all moved out of my father's house and were living within a few miles of one another. We hung out together in a way that was unusual for other siblings I knew at the time. Joe and Paul, Mary's fiancé, were in a band together and we would hang around her house while the band and other musician friends would jam.

In early spring Mary reported these funny red spots on her legs and said she was bruising easily. We were leaving a matinee when she told me she would get really tired whenever she rode her bicycle lately and she was planning to see a doctor about it. In a month we knew she had leukemia. In six months she was at Stanford University hospital in Palo Alto, California, undergoing chemotherapy. In seven months, she was gone.

It doesn't seem that I've been 100% healthy a day since. I started having terrifying panic attacks shortly after Mary's death, but no one could tell me what they were and what was wrong with me. I had never heard of a panic attack. I sank into depression from the frequent, sudden bursts of terror and the emotional 'hangover' they would produce. Four years later I was watching Phil Donahue's talk show and they were speaking about agoraphobia, where people experience panic away from the safety of their homes. I felt a profound recognition of what they were saying. I called someone who called someone and soon I was seeing a psychologist and taking anti-depressant medication. She would later diagnose me with chronic Post Traumatic Stress Disorder (PTSD). Watching my beloved sister die had threatened a very tenuous sense of safety, order and trust I felt in the world.

Between 1979 and the spring of 1988—when I first felt ill—I had gotten married, and Keith and I had bought our first home. My career was evolving in directions I had never imagined and I had lots of wonderful friends. The panic and depression had resolved with the medication I had been prescribed.

When this sudden onset of flu-like symptoms appeared, the psychologist—who I hadn't seen since stabilizing on the Pamelor a few years earlier—suspected that the anti-depressant had reached toxic levels in my blood and was responsible for my poor health. Even though tests showed that my blood levels of the drug were normal, she said that what are considered to be therapeutic levels for most people can be toxic for some. The way I was having trouble finding words made her very suspicious that this was the case. So I stopped taking the Pamelor. It didn't make any difference.

Still ill and feeling so discouraged and despairing that no answers would be forthcoming, I was unable to see any other alternative but to return to work. My job offered a lot of flexibility and the day wasn't too long. I had been working in that position for so long that I could do it with my eyes closed. These things helped me to be able to return, but any other activity aside from that job fell by the wayside. I went to work, went home and to bed. The next day, same thing. Weekends I would be so sick and tired I couldn't do my ordinary chores let alone a little recreation.

I began to see an acupuncturist who was entirely sympathetic and eager to help me. Western medicine treats the symptoms of CFS, since it does not yet identify an underlying cause. Chinese medicine, on the other hand, does identify underlying cause(s), they just aren't in terms that we Westerners understand.

I was pleasantly surprised at how refreshing and relaxing the acupuncture treatments were and I enjoyed them, but I felt that I was not improving in any substantial way. I knew little about alternative forms of medicine at the time and was very westernized in my expectations. I was used to a quick fix. With no prior experience that taught me to have confidence in more subtle therapies, and little energy available for dragging myself to appointments, I discontinued.

I also tried homeopathy during this time. The homeopathist was recommended by my good friend, Carol, and I liked her. Her office was chunky with hippie furniture in primary colors and had a thoughtful play area for waiting children. I was pretty open-minded about trying unfamiliar forms of health care and was impressed that mothers trusted their children to this form of healing. I figured that the people who grew up in cultures where these modalities were more the norm had just as much trouble putting their faith in the Western approach to healthcare as we did to understanding theirs. It's all relative, I guess.

After a lengthy history and examination, the homeopathist mixed up an herbal remedy for me to take. Homeopathy is based on the premise that like cures like. I was warned that I would likely feel worse before I felt better. And so I did. So much worse that I felt I had to stop. At this point I was so frightened by my intense discomfort and the not-knowing where it all came from that I was unable to trust that we were helping and not hurting. I chose to retreat and went home licking my wounds. Today I understand that they call that period of worsening a "healing crisis" and that it is a common, although not a certain, event in the recovery process. All I knew then was that my goal was to go in the other direction; to feel *better*, not worse.

Soon after that my friend, Daphne, who was visiting from Arizona speculated, "Maybe you have that chronic fatigue disease that's been on the news." I hadn't heard about this and asked her what she knew, but she had nothing else, just that it sounded similar to what I was desribing. I was getting used to people suggesting cures and comparing me to others that they knew or had heard of: "My neighbor has a cousin who had the same symptoms that you do. She took this vitamin powder and was completely cured!" or, "Have you tried bee pollen? My aunt was feeling tired all the time and she started taking it and is back to normal. She swears by it. It's worth a try. What have you got to lose?" Trained medical professionals had gone through their entire repertoire to no avail. So, I let Daphne's comment about a new fatigue disease sink to the back of my mind.

After another six months, I left my long-held and beloved teaching position for good—admitting utter defeat. I thought that if I had nothing to do it wouldn't matter so much that I *couldn't* do anything. I had given up on a diagnosis, resigning myself to the flu-aches and myriad other symptoms of "unknown origin." My plan was to work part-time and at my own pace as a consultant to special education teachers and programs, helping with curriculum, licensing and language-skill building. I got a position immediately and found the more flexible schedule to be easier. I also found that without a set schedule to adhere to, I was taking more sick days (but without the sick leave pay) and therefore our finances were suffering. I was choosing to stay at home more often than go out to work or promote myself. Every day was a struggle just to get out of bed. My body wanted to sleep twelve hours a night and still couldn't seem to refresh itself for the next day. It was just so hard to force myself up and out without anyone expecting me to show up somewhere.

That first consulting position had flexible hours and was close to my home. I was there for six months. When it ended I needed to put more effort into marketing myself. I was getting work, but it was just so difficult to stay motivated and to push myself, dragging my aching, feverish and exhausted body all over town for appointments. I worked less and less, allowing myself to take more days off than Keith and I could afford—and feeling guilty about it.

Feeling defeated once again, I went back to full-time work in special education as a vocational counselor. We needed the income and I needed the schedule to force me to get going each day. And besides, I reasoned that if I wasn't going to be getting any better, I just had to learn to live with—and work with—this thing. I had begun to have occasional days where I felt at least halfway human. Maybe I was adjusting with time, integrating the fatigue and aches into my "normal" state and learning to function in spite of it.

I continued off and on to seek medical help, but was mostly discouraged and began to feel it was a waste of my time and money. Things can get rather costly, especially when you are looking outside of the Western medical model where most tests, procedures and remedies are not covered by health insurance. I would usually go for a spell ignoring doctors altogether, frustrated with their inability to tell me what was going on. It was so obvious to me that my body had some disease. And I came to believe over time that staying away from doctors and their treatments may have been one of the reasons I eventually recovered to the degree that I did. Not only was I wearing myself out physically and emotionally with all of those appointments, tests and ineffective treatments, but they also took time away from resting and facing my emotional and spiritual self, where I thought I might have a chance to learn to help myself cope. Endless medical appointments were a way of feeding the illusion that there was some great wizard with all the answers hiding behind the next curtain while I myself was powerless.

I could tell the doctors were getting tired of me, too. They didn't seem to like cases they couldn't solve. If it weren't for my 99.4 degree fever, I am sure they would have sent me off to therapy and washed their hands of me completely. The thought that this could all be "in my head" was a scary one to me, almost equally as frightening as considering a physical cause. Could my mind really make up the aches, the cough, the pain in my feet? Why would it? And how could I stop it if it was unconscious?

One internist I saw had mentioned something called "Chronic Fatigue Syndrome" rather under her breath and as a last resort possibility. I had tested weakly positive for mononucleosis twice. When all the testing had been done (and all the king's horses and all the king's men couldn't put me back together again!) I asked very tentatively if it was time to consider this chronic fatigue thing she had spoken about a few appointments back, but she acted a bit appalled and said she would want to do more tests before she would be comfortable with that diagnosis. By now I was so tired of blood tests, urine tests, drinking-funny-concoctions-and-seeing-what-happens tests. I just couldn't do it. I was beat.

I had been seeing mostly specialists thus far and decided to go see my usual family doctor to suggest to him the idea of the chronic fatigue disease and see what he had to say. He told me that it simply didn't exist, it was a crock. He presented a thick medical volume from which he proceeded to copy me several pages of text on some disease where you suffered paralysis on one side of the face. Myasthenia Gravis, I think it was. He thought I more closely fit the symptom picture for that, alerted, I guess, by the intermittent facial numbness I was having, and he proceeded to order tests. I went home and read the description. It didn't sound anything like me. It was at about that point that I quit putting any hope in medicine.

By then I was learning how to live with so much discomfort and so little energy, doing everything in steps and in the shortest time possible. Sometimes just lugging the heavy vacuum cleaner out of the closet and into the living room took all of my reserves for that day. It might not be until two or three more days had passed before I had the stamina to plug it in, turn it on and push it around. It's important to note that I included the step of plugging in the vacuum cleaner. It amplifies that one tiny step and illustrates how big it becomes when you are ill and fatigued. I shopped at the nearest grocery store, even if a better one was just another half a mile away. This need to economize on energy was something very difficult for others to understand. I would take every shortcut, many that would sound ridiculous to people if they knew. Like leaving my hairbrush on the bathroom counter rather than storing it in a nearby drawer just so I wouldn't have to go through those extra steps to get it out. We ate instant and convenience foods even though I was a pretty health conscious vegetarian. Even still, I would prepare the evening meal in steps beginning early in the day so I would expend less effort and could renew my energy in between. I'd get the pots I would be using out in the morning and set them in their places on the stovetop. Early in the afternoon I'd do the prep work like peeling and chopping. That way, by evening I could manage getting dinner made because so much of the work was already done. Something as small as reaching for a pan and lifting it out of the cupboard often took more than I could muster. Keith arrived home from work many days to hear me say I couldn't manage dinner, did he mind going for take-out?

Some time went by before I was to look again to the medical profession for an answer. I managed to work at my job in spite of my constant tiredness and body aches, but would collapse during my down time and I had no other life to speak of. I toughed it out on my own, desperately looking for a formula or a key that would restore my former health. By this time I had heard a little more about the fatigue disease. I knew it was called "Chronic Fatigue Syndrome," or CFS. I learned that its standing as a medical condition was controversial and, as I had already discovered, many doctors didn't believe it was real. I became severely depressed, struggling and coaching myself to rise above it, even while I ached from head to toe and feared for my future.

Journal Entry, September 3, 1990:

This is the plan I have put together to free me from the rut of my life with THE FLU THAT NEVER ENDS:

Housework—try to keep up. Do what I can every day and then see if Keith will help catch up on the weekends. I recognize that a clean house is important to my sense of comfort but I need to learn to relax some of this.

Work—keep a light attitude.

Social—stay in touch in whatever way I can. Focus on giving in reachable ways: notes and letters, compliments, phone calls.

Spirit—read, watch the seasons, keep the faerie light alive in my heart.

Health—eat well, sleep well, exercise as much as I can tolerate, visualize and use daily affirmations. Rest extra when needed. Take sick days! Say no when I want to whether I feel bad or not. Stay away from sickness thoughts. Concentrate on the positive. Pray.

I was finding it harder and harder to relate to people who had the energy for children, career, health clubs *and* a social life. I watched people sprint across the street through traffic and couldn't even begin to locate a source for that kind of energy burst inside myself. I knew I used to be able to run, but could not even fathom the mechanics of it anymore. I worried, "What if I *had* to run from something? I wouldn't be able to. I'd have to succumb." I still had no name for the condition that took away my full, exciting life and replaced it with this nothingness.

I remember putting so much pressure on myself, feeling like I wasn't measuring up. I had healthy friends who were meditating every day, working out, keeping up a house, working full-time jobs, and so on. I had desires of my own. I wanted to finish college and do volunteer work. I wanted a hobby and to find a type of exercise I could love. My adorable golden retriever, KC, who I was goofy in love with, needed walking and brushing and, in fact, all of the critters in my household needed to be fed a couple of times a day, husband included. I had an incredibly sweet new nephew whom I wanted to spend great amounts of lovely time with. I was seeing less and less of friends. I wanted so badly to have the energy for all of these people and things.

My symptoms had begun to vary a bit. In spite of my tiredness it was difficult to fall asleep at night. Each morning I would give myself time to wake up and then evaluate my level of pain, mental fogginess and energy. At this point in my illness, I could often get through a day at work without too much misery. Mostly

I worked at my desk and sat in meetings. I rarely could manage any more than that. And when the fatigue would come on really strong and I could barely lift my head off the pillow, I never knew if it would last an hour, a day, a week, or months. Each time my symptoms would abate to a discernable degree and then return, I was afraid all over again that they would last forever. During this time I never felt healthy like my old self—I certainly wasn't well by normal standards and most days were not what I had begun to call my "good" days.

I kept hearing more and more about CFS and was reading related magazine articles with great curiosity. I didn't know anyone, even indirectly, with this syndrome. Long before the Centers for Disease Control (CDC) figured out how to define CFS, I had become progressively more certain that it was what I had. The personal stories I was reading rang so true. I wasn't particularly thrilled to have something many doctors believed was just hysteria, hypochondriasis, or depression. But I knew in my heart and in my body that it wasn't these things—*couldn't be*. I yearned to have a name for what was wrong with me so the not-knowing could be over and I could get on with whatever came next. Anything to move out of this ongoing emptiness....

In 1992, I read about a Dr. Jay Goldstein in Beverly Hills, California. He ran a place called the Chronic Fatigue Syndrome Institute. I lived just three hours north of his clinic, in the blue-skied coastal city of San Luis Obispo, and decided it was worth big-city doctor money to go to someone who could finally tell me if this is what I had or not. He believed it was real, was researching it, had lots of patients who had it. I figured that if anyone would know CFS when they saw it, it was him.

Keith kindly drove me to my appointment, as there was no way I could manage to get there on my own. Not only was I too depleted and sleepy, but I had begun to find that driving on freeways and in busy traffic felt way too over-stimulating. There was just too much to track and my brain felt like it would explode or blow a fuse. When I tried to merge into traffic, I felt I couldn't gauge the distance between cars in the brief time that I had to look away from the road in front of me to change lanes. Being anywhere unfamiliar just amplified things and I just didn't feel able to keep myself safe when I drove.

The very day we went to the Chronic Fatigue Institute I got my diagnosis—indeed I had CFS. At last I had something with a name. All of my symptoms made sense in the context of CFS. In fact, I had two somethings. After poking around my shoulders and neck at some very painful points Dr. Goldstein said that I also had something called Fibromyalgia (FMS) and that's what was causing the migratory pain I experienced. I cried with gratefulness, feeling foolish and fearing that the doctor would think I was malingering after all if I expressed joy at such a diagnosis, but he said it was a common response, the end (beginning?) of a long emotional journey for many. The effort and emotion of that trip cost me several days in bed but it was absolutely worth it.

At the time, the diagnosis was welcome. The not-knowing had caused me so much fear. And other people want to know what's wrong with you, too. This was my proof that I wasn't making it up, pitiful as that sounds. I wasn't focused on the fact that there was no cure and that the "C" in CFS stands for *chronic*. I was just relieved to know it wasn't something that could kill me. And when I learned that it could go away, I hung onto that as best I could.

My diagnosis helped me to end the cycle of fear that comes with undiagnosed chronic illness and put some closure on my many heretofore unanswered questions. Going directly to a specialist can save thousands of dollars otherwise spent on ineffective treatments, inconclusive medical tests and office visit charges.

Where did the CFS come from? I fit the profile that many specialists have proposed: highly active and in good health prior to a sudden onset, a connection to polio via my mother who entered the hospital with it shortly after my birth and I was also one of the recipients of the first live polio vaccines, a history of depression and anxiety and early childhood trauma. These were statistically significant, but no one could yet say the cause, or causes, of CFS.

Dr. Goldstein suggested a couple of tests from which he found common results in other CFS patients. I tested positive for both: an in-office hyperventilation test and a 24-hour urine collection to test for *spuma virus*. These tests were state-of-the-art at the time. He suggested I try taking malic acid (found where nutritional supplements are sold) and Zantac (yes, the heartburn medicine that is now available over the counter) along with a very minute dose of Elavil, an antidepressant, to help me to sleep at night. Dr. Goldstein explained that people with CFS commonly respond to medications at doses far below what is considered to be the therapeutic level. At the higher, usual dosages they tend to experience too many side effects. He seemed to know so much about CFS. I felt euphoric to be talking to someone who could finally help me, someone who understood my language. None of my symptoms or stories surprised him. My relief was palpable. My hope renewed.

For the next blessed several months I thought I might be cured. The malic acid/Zantac combination had been fairly miraculous for me. Within a few weeks of my appointment with Dr. Goldstein, I noticed I had more energy than I had felt in a very long time. I hadn't attempted to resume my pre-illness activity level, but after a month and a half I started to wonder if the CFS was gone.

I had just been through four years of sickness, pain and despair. I felt like I had found my Mighty Oz behind the curtain and was granted my life back. After about seven months, I thought it was over, the CFS was in my past and I didn't need to take the pills anymore. Hadn't I read somewhere that four years was the average length of time people were sick with CFS?

I quit taking the medications and relapsed within a week. Right back where I was before my visit with Oz in the Emerald City, paralyzed and sleepy in the enchanted poppy field. I quickly reinstated my regimen but it appeared that I had lost the initial momentum and the pills now had no effect, which I was to learn is common with CFS.

I felt enormous disappointment and retreated, utterly defeated. I could practically hear the CFS snickering at me. In retrospect, I had just experienced my first real remission/relapse cycle. I don't think it was a coincidence that the remission occurred while following Dr. Goldstien's treatment. The placebo effect does not last that long. And I've since seen malic acid repeatedly on lists of the most effective treatments for CFS. It was a real lesson for me. From that point on I would remit and relapse many times, though my remissions would rarely be as symptom-free or as long-lasting as that glorious first time.

Two

"The Chinese sage Lao Tzu tells us that the usefulness of things is in their emptiness. The useful part of the wheel is the hub; the useful part of a pot is the empty space within."

—Laurence G. Boldt, Zen and the Art of Making a Living

I began to see a counselor to help me with the depression that seeped all over everything: my sense of belonging, of value, my marriage and my role within it. My job, social life, spirit, home and family. The pain, frustration and coming to terms with so much loss. I began to think of people with CFS like myself as the living dead.

One of the more sensible things that came out of the therapy was that I was encouraged to again take a leave of absence from my job. I had been getting increasingly sick and depressed about the situation at work. There was some struggle with personalities and major dysfunction—*what? In the workplace?*—that was stressing me to the point that my health was paying a big price. The stress that my illness created in my life was more than enough for me to manage. When I compounded that with job-related stress, I wasn't coping well. My therapist had introduced me to a wonderful local doctor, Steve Clarke, who validated so much of my experience and consulted with Dr. Goldstein in Beverly Hills regarding my care. I felt endlessly grateful to him. After several appointments, at which I broke down sobbing with despair, he strongly suggested a three month leave of absence from work and wrote it out as a prescription for me to show my employer.

With both my doctor and my counselor telling me my health would only continue to suffer if I didn't eliminate the major stressor—my job—I got the message. The thought of not working was hard for me to bear. It was the only remnant of my former life I had; my only lifeline into the 'real' world where people went about their daily business, hurrying around, everything urgent and of the utmost importance.

It wasn't until I considered the need to give up working that I realized what I really feared: that *I* might disappear with it. Who was I if I wasn't doing these things? *Was* I if I wasn't doing these things? And where's the value in the me collapsed on the sofa? I couldn't see how Keith and I could manage on one income and I resisted putting us in that position, fearing my own guilt and projections of resentment. Reminding myself every few minutes that this was just temporary, I hauled myself into the director's office at work, showed her my note from Dr. Clarke and then went home.

In such a busy world we forget how to be still. When I stopped going to work I had a real struggle with the nothingness that was there to replace it. Ways-to-fill-your-life had its place but ways-to-be-empty was certainly the greater struggle for me. There was a sense of shutting down: the factory is closed. My sense of my own worth was utterly challenged as feelings of uselessness grew with the necessary surrender to my illness.

I found it hard to resist the urge to fill the empty hours. I set about looking for ways I could be useful. Within a week I was volunteering to work with abused children and registering for classes in childhood play therapy at a university ninety miles from my home. I finally had the time to do what I really wanted. It was hard to resist. The part of me that lived in my head and liked going ninety miles per hour pursuing a myriad of causes and interests remained, but my body refused to comply. Within another couple of weeks I realized that I really couldn't schedule anything at all and I quit the volunteer work and the school. No longer able to count on my health enough to make commitments, I began the long hard road to finding value and fulfillment living a physically passive life.

My self-judgement was relentless. How could I allow myself to do nothing when I felt I needed to rest? Isn't that called "laziness?" What is valuable about me if I am not contributing, participating, living? What is there to take pride in? How do I live with feeling useless?

At some level I recognized that in order to get well enough to be active again, I needed to learn to find contentment in the quiet time with myself and try to break free of the idea that my life was "on hold." It's easy to feel like you're just in a waiting phase and that this somehow isn't the real thing. But years were going by and I wasn't getting well. If this wasn't my real life, I was truly lost—miles and miles and miles from home. In the ultimate failure of my denial and resistance, I had at last come to the place where I knew I needed to make myself a home in the landscape I had been so desperate to deny. I closed my eyes and clicked my heels together. "There's no place like home."

Those of us living with chronic illness must reach for the place where we can see that the emptiness isn't empty after all. We are full of the nature and spirit that makes us individuals. We are full of the very thing that those who have chosen to be close to us love. And that is where the living happens. It might require a shift in perspective to appreciate. In the stillness of there being nothing, we can come to see the vastness of ourselves that is something. And when we take hold of the something that is there in the emptiness, like lifting a smooth shell off the beach, that is when we take our first step to discovering what's really behind the curtain and we can begin to live our life in the moment we are in.

Letter to my Doctor, June, 1993:

Dear Dr. Clarke,

I wanted to write to inform you that I have stopped attending school. It was a very hard decision for me to make and I wanted to tell you something about it.

I realize that my life needs to be about getting well right now. It is time to heal. I made that commitment when I took leave from my job. And I see that I have been afraid that there is no vocational future for me. An education seemed like a timely opportunity that eased my concern. But I came to know that it was purely a fear reaction that helped me to visualize a future so that it didn't look so empty and scary to me.

I could see that my drive was getting the better of me again. The rest and quiet that I need and the holding off on living is very hard to deal with. It has occurred to me that what is necessary is surrendering and learning to be comfortable just being alone with myself and with what is at this moment.

School was already making me sicker after just two sessions of a weekly class. I began feeling that settled-in tiredness and resignation I had felt when working. I found myself sacrificing in other areas of my life to accommodate school. I was allocating the little energy I had—to fix a meal, take a short walk, brush my dog—to my internal demand that I be someone who is productive. I saw that I was flip-flopping my priorities again.

I am trying hard to accept that right now has to be about getting well and that when I am well, I will get to the next thing. I must relinquish concern for what and when the next step will be and learn to stay with this moment right now, trusting my future to the generosity of the universe.

Our expectations that we must always be "doing" to have value is unfair. We have no trouble seeing the value in a newborn infant or in the person sitting next to us. It's when we turn to apply it to ourselves that it doesn't seem to hold up.

It has been speculated many times that the people who get CFS are "over-achievers." I believe it is this same tendency to seek proof of our value as people that compels us to produce so much tangible evidence of it. With CFS—and the stripping of our ability to produce—we come face-to-face with our naked selves, giving us ample opportunity to examine such internalized beliefs. When we get into the trap of thinking of this ill time as an unfortunate detour and derailment of our life, we miss the bigger picture and can make ourselves miserable with guilt and feelings of uselessness.

In my own behavior I could see how much I needed to feel useful. Not just any old useful, but useful in a people-helping way. I wanted to make a difference. I didn't know how to do that anymore.

At one time I had loved my job. I certainly didn't love some of the challenges and dysfunctional interrelationships, but I loved what it was that I did and I felt that I had been called to special education for the last seventeen years. This time I took three months off to rest and when I found myself no better physically but way better emotionally, I didn't look back. I had moved through resistance and denial, at least for now. I would re-visit them in the future, because lessons are not learned once, but many times—and Chronic Fatigue Syndrome is an *ocean* of lessons. Symptoms ebb and flow. Coping ebbs and flows. Like the pain, the epiphany is migratory.

With the support of my doctor I went on state disability, which I was eligible for through my job. I also began the application process for Social Security Disability benefits since I had been warned that this process would take several months. I was fortunate to get state benefits immediately and to have the Social Security Disability process go smoothly.

Most people I know who have CFS have had to appeal a denial of their disability claim with Social Security. The process takes months or even years, and is very stressful. It creates an interesting conflict in the applicant who must prove they are too ill to function productively, leaving little energy or incentive to try to get better until the process is complete.

My claim was accepted on the first try. Dr. Clarke had been able to submit a letter giving great detail about my limitations since I had shared them with him throughout my visits. In addition, the Social Security Administration had directed me to see a doctor they had appointed who said I was a "textbook case of CFS."

Three

Journal Entry, September 14, 1993:

Tension & Relaxation

Tension

flies like

a misfolded paper airplane,

crashing,

thundering,

reckless.

Relaxation

glides over

waves of slippery water.

Journal Entry September 20, 1993:

Very confused, panicked, depressed today. I am so frightened. I'm not sure why. Life feels so meaningless. I can't stand the thought of doing nothing. There must be something sunny and exciting that I can do. But I can hardly move most days. I can't keep any kind of schedule (therapy is the only thing on the calendar). How can I have value if I do nothing? How can I be interesting? This is too boring and working on my inner self is too scary. I have lost my momentum absolutely at this point. Is there no turning back? I want to row in a boat on a quiet river, walk along a country path, create things, learn things, make money and spend it. I want all of this but can't pull the effort out of myself. Why did I have to get this stupid illness? I realize that in the fourteen years since Mary died I've had two major surgeries, panic disorder, and CFS. Always before that it was just colds and flu. Simple stuff. What's going on? I'm remembering that moment in the hospital during Mary's chemotherapy when she said she was so tired of feeling awful sick and she just wanted to die, that she didn't care about anything anymore but being relieved of her pain and nausea. I am peeking into that memory and feel I can actually relate to her tiredness. Tired of the fight. Tired of the discomfort. Estranged from ordinary life.

For the first several years of my illness, much of my time was spent in a cave of denial, refusing to hear the creaks and moans of my body and trying to carry on with my life as though nothing had changed, really. When denial didn't work—for obvious reasons—resistance would often take its place. If I just kept pushing…. If I pretended hard that the CFS wasn't there. If I took this pill or avoided that food. If I hated it enough I could annihilate it. One day, I knew, the doctors would find out what was *really* wrong with me and fix it.

Eventually I began looking more inward. There must be some work I can do to help myself, I thought, some way to stop this. I kept running an analogy through my mind of dumping out a sock drawer to clean it out. Carefully evaluating each pair for holes, comfort, do I really like the color? Do I ever wear these? This is something I did occasionally in my real life, with my actual socks. I wouldn't put a sock back in the drawer until I was sure it still had value to me.

In my analogy, these "socks" became the things of my life; the people, the habits, the job, the diet. Each must be scrutinized. I examined each item and asked, does this support my healing? I set out to consciously make my life about things that felt good and nurturing. I kept very light exercise for instance, as I found that it helped with the pain and left me feeling more movable. I embraced and welcomed as much of nature as I could get in the form of walks in the woods, gardening, or sitting in a lazy lawn chair reading a book in the green of my yard. I paid attention to the mental boost that certain music gave me and made sure I listened frequently. These things went back into the drawer.

What went out? Inviting people to dinner out of a sense of obligation. Stressing over the crazy interrelationships at work, now in my past. Forcing myself to keep up with housework when I felt too weak. Thinking that I had no value if I wasn't contributing something. Hanging on to relationships that didn't work thinking I had the power to change or control them. Doing favors for people because I was afraid they wouldn't like me if I said no.

In went nutritional supplementation and an answering machine to screen telephone calls; out, too much responsibility. In, an ear to hear my body and permission to give it rest when it asked. (If I was just about to get in the car to go somewhere and suddenly became aware that I didn't really want to go, I got out of the car and stayed home.) Out went lists of things to do that only fed my unhealthy drive to accomplish at all costs and led to a sense of failure if I couldn't complete the list. Out went anything written in stone. All plans became tentative.

For a long time I had been observing that the things that worked for me were not doctor's medicines or expensive treatments. So many ways to approach healthcare, many not covered by insurance and expensive for someone who wasn't working. It was hard to be patient for treatments that worked on a more subtle level. I had begun to notice that the things that seemed to help me were free or nearly so. Things like resting, eating nutritious foods, listening to music that lifted my mood, following a sleep schedule. I decided to stop stressing so much over trying to find—and pay for—a treatment that would cure me and instead paid attention to the things that were right before me. Chasing a cure can be just another form of resistance, after all. I found it to be costly monetarily, physically and emotionally. And with years of illness to look back on, I could see that it hadn't made enough of a difference for me. I still felt sick, was still in pain, still depressed and scared. And so was everybody else I met with CFS regardless of their pills, appointments, machines and manipulations. I knew intuitively that the work of getting well lay elsewhere for me.

As I proceeded to reorder the contents of my life and left the search for a medical cure to others, I began to find some kind of peace in my days. The more my drawer (life) filled with supportive, nurturing experiences, the more I seemed to heal. Encouraged, I continued to evaluate the stuff of my life and to constantly question how I was living in relation to my illness.

It's easy to sink into feeling like a victim and to believe you are powerless when you so abruptly lose your health. The act of re-ordering my life brought lovely choice back into the equation. It is vital to our well-being to be able to see where there is choice.

Some time after I had quit my job and gone on Social Security Disability, I was walking in a local park and suddenly felt a great sense of euphoria. I had become aware that I was walking through this lovely park with friendly trees and the birds and squirrels in the middle of a day when most people were at work. I wasn't struggling at a job trying to please a lot of other people who didn't care about me. I was with flowers! I took a deep breath and felt my lungs fill with a new joy and peace. I didn't need to continuously kick myself and feel like I was failing because I couldn't seem to pick myself up off the floor and do something useful. It was at that moment I stopped fretting over not being able to work.

I saw how my life had been missing this slow and lazy side and how I had needed to learn to balance work with leisure. Even though I didn't need to look far or hard to notice my aches and fever, I didn't feel at all like complaining.

What a gift! I saw how beauty could share space with CFS. Encouraged by this experience, I was able to shift some of my attention away from my discomfort and notice what was good. Moments like this began to multiply and gratitude became a familiar feeling to me.

I first encountered the idea that resisting something simply makes it worse in Erhard Seminars Training (EST) in 1970. EST was originally an intensive three-day weekend workshop in self-awareness, very popular in the early seventies. We were led through many examples of resistance over the course of the weekend like, what happens when you try not to think of someone or something? It makes it grow.

EST taught me a lot of things that would come in handy during this period of my life, some two decades later. I recall very clearly one of the earlier exercises of the training where the audience was invited to call out what causes headaches. People replied with things like solving complicated math problems, screaming children, fog, hot dogs, going without your morning cup of coffee, the smell of dirty diapers, sitting too close to the television, crossing your eyes. The trainers wrote these and dozens of others on a huge blackboard on the stage. The only one of these I personally could relate to was hot dogs. Many I thought were ridiculous. At the end of this exercise it was clear that an individual's own expectations could be as responsible for the headache as any true biological phenomenon.

On the day of my walk in the park I suddenly "got" how that same concept of resistance and expectation can apply to illness. I saw how, in making an enemy out of CFS, I was making an enemy out of my own body. The harder I said "no" and resisted my condition, the louder it responded. Just like all the times I decided not to eat chocolate anymore, and then chocolate was all I could think about. It was clear that my walk in the park could have been about how much my ankles hurt, how cold it was outside and the discomfort of my allergies just as easily as it could be about accepting the beauty in that moment. It's where I put my attention and how I either reject or embrace what I find that makes the difference.

Of course, I was not, from that day forward, a happy-go-lucky person. We don't get better in a straight line. I continued to have "bad" days, but tried not to look at them as something to fight or regret and began instead to allow my body the rest it required. There was no hurry to get anything done, no need to feel I failed or to add any pressure. I avoided making firm commitments to myself and others and was consciously learning to take the time to just be good to myself. I knew that the CFS wasn't going to kill me and I was able to release the apprehension that another shoe might yet drop. As I relaxed around that awareness, I could see that it was time to focus on the parts of me that *did* work and learn to live in a different way, without attaching any thought that *different* was "bad" or "less-than." I could see how my physical experience was being exacerbated by things that were under my control like my attitude toward myself and perceptions about my health and its impact and power over me. If I could learn to move my focus away from how sick I felt, I thought I might be happier. That sounds very simple and, in fact, in some ways it is just that simple.

I often look back at this re-ordering, the sock drawer period and my walk-in-the-woods awakening, as a launch into my healing phase. Once I had opened the door to such introspection I found that I had access to incredible, wonderful, heartful revelations that made me feel powerful in direct contrast to my physical weakness. Being able to hear my own voice after forty years of intense drive to please others was a challenge. But the more I listened—I figured I had all the time in the world—the easier it got and the things that I heard taught me invaluable lessons about my own inner connection to Spirit and the abundance of miracles therein.

This work led me right up to the Mighty Oz behind the curtain I had drawn around my psyche, and here I found my own hands on the controls. I realized that, as so many wise people have said, many of the answers were right there inside me all along. My search for wellness via a wizard or a magic pill had been an illusion that had kept me from seeing the truth of my own power. I have come to believe that the key to healing, the mighty Oz if you will, lies in accessing this inner landscape where the heart touches and knows its true nature. Here, all is pure and detached from the "shoulds" we tend to pile on ourselves. It felt like I was reclaiming my life. The challenge, as always, was to integrate the epiphany in such a way that I could hang on to its blessings, especially in the hardest times.

Have you ever played the computer game, *Myst?* The answer to each clue is just a step towards the next clue. As you move through the game you have to hold all the previous answers in your head to stay on your course towards the ultimate resolution of the riddle. Of course, with the cognitive interference of CFS, this is very challenging. I kept having to go back and re-visit clues I'd already solved so that everything could keep making sense to me. Though definitely not as graphically interesting as the game, chronic illness runs a similar course. I learned something. I forgot it. I went back and re-learned it. But I felt a gradual progress of sorts.

Four

Journal Entry, March 18, 1994:

<u>Precursors/Predictors</u>

- *alarm clock/early or rushed mornings set up a tired day*

- *open doors/windows or being outside brings on severe allergy symptoms any time of the year*

- *damp, cold weather brings chills, aches, fatigue, fever, swollen glands. May actually be changes in weather or barometric pressure rather than damp & cold, or both.*

- *over 2 hours of activity takes a half day to 2 days to recover from*

- *family/friends visiting counts as activity!!!*

- *caffeine anytime = insomnia*

- *menses wipes out for 2–3 days*

- *perfume strips in magazines bother my eyes/sinuses*

- *fresh mowed grass = allergies*

- *cigarette smoke, perfume, fumes of any kind bother my eyes and sinus and may trigger relapse*

- *stress makes everything worse*

<u>Program</u>

- *avoid sugar, caffeine, additives*

- *yoga*

- *do half of what you feel up to*

- *learn to say no*

- *avoid chemicals, fumes, smoke*

- *take vitamins*

- *keep a journal*

- *get plenty of sleep*

- *drink lots of filtered water*

- *meditate*

- *breathe*

- *no cocoa, chocolate after 6pm*

- *naps*

Curious to see what a support group might have to offer, I went to a meeting for people with CFS/FMS and met some wonderful friends there. I had, by now, read the few personal stories of people living with CFS that had been published, and I regularly received journals in the mail that were dedicated to the self-help movement that had begun to grow as patients searched for answers and were not finding them in the medical community. Aside from the relief of being with people who could totally understand what I was experiencing, I learned a great deal from observing others with a chronic illness. I started to see unconscious behaviors and attitudes that might keep a person stuck in the murky waters of CFS that I could not have seen in myself without their example. I found a lot of people who were unable to say no, who helped others at their own expense, people just like me who pushed themselves to be productive and fell into despair when they were unable to sustain the effort. People who spent all of their time and conversation on how bad they felt. People with no hope, no power.

Having not quite figured out where to go with my observations, I was still focused on the outward things that I could do to help myself and had begun to develop a bit of a regimen to support my healing. Routines had to be altered, and frequently were, based on my current level of functioning which could change from day to day and even hour to hour. I attempted to retain at least some physical activity. This was, perhaps, my formerly thin self feeling reluctant about the weight I was gaining more than any thought of reducing pain or improving strength. Sometimes I could manage a half-block walk, other times I was doing laps with a kickboard at the pool at the YMCA.

Sleep regulation seemed necessary and perhaps the most vital of all. I got into the habit of going to bed and getting up at the same time every day. Even if I found myself unable to go to sleep, I stayed in bed figuring the rest was beneficial even if I was just lying still with closed eyes. Dr. Goldstein had prescribed a small dose of Elavil (0.5 mg) to help with sleep, but I could never really tell a difference. Perhaps it helped me to sleep a little deeper, once I did manage to doze off.

Journal Entry, May 1, 1994:

Nurturing All of Me:

Physical: take warm baths, go for walks, eat healthy, get good sleep, yoga, garden, rest.

Emotional: therapy, write letters, journal, read, watch funny television shows, time with friends

Mental: read, write, watch public television, crosswords, learn about health

Spiritual: nature walks, read, meditate, music, garden, sing, art, visualize

---

I usually took some form of vitamin or herbal supplement, but never really went wild with this like many people I came to know with CFS or fibromyalgia. I just couldn't spend the money and I didn't see that any of those other people were doing all that well anyway. I was also aware that there was no one treatment that was successful on a significant percentage of those who tried it. I saw many different things working and not working for many different people. With one it was colon cleansing. With another, homeopathy. For some, raw foods. What made one well, might make another sicker or have no impact. Does this mean the treatments themselves have no intrinsic power, I wondered? Does it point to the biological differences in each of us or in the power of faith? Is it the modality or what one believes that's important? No one cure. Many things working to some degree. Nothing working for everyone. Hmm.

I figured that if something was discovered that was successful enough for me to warrant spending the money and risking side effects and whatever else, it was going to be on the cover of *Newsweek* and we'd all be reading about it. Nonetheless, from time to time I would hear or read about something that sounded sensible and I would try it for a spell. This would always be short-lived as I would either experience uncomfortable side effects or would not notice any benefit. *I came to believe that the best thing I could do for FM and CFS was easy and free: get fresh air, reduce my exposure to toxic substances, really rest, eat healthy foods, find lots of joy (music, nature), have honest dialogue with my psyche, get some exercise, drink lots of clean water, and don't spend all of my time thinking about how sick I feel. Focus on the good. Remain aware of the ways in which I talk to myself. Find the place that lies between resistance and resignation. Recognize the teacher and pay attention to the lessons.*

I'm very suspicious about toxins. Many hold the theory that they play a great part in sustaining CFS—maybe even play a part in the cause. It makes sense to me that anyone who is not well might want to pay attention to the level of exposure to toxic substances in their life. For myself, I decided to identify and eliminate as many as I possibly could. I can picture my body as a vase or other receptacle with a limited capacity. My body seems to have a particular threshold of tolerance and when I overflow with chemical exposure, my symptoms worsen. I had seen this happen many times. So if I take some control and lower my exposure as much as I (as an individual) can, then maybe there will be room for the exposure I can't control without overflowing into symptoms.

One of the ways that I reduced my exposure was to invest in a water filter and use it for everything from water in which to wash and cook our foods to drinking water. We installed filters on the showerheads after I had read somewhere how hot water, and thus, steam is a carrier of many substances that may be in the water. We buy organic produce and eat as low on the food chain as possible. I wear natural fiber clothes. I quit wearing perfume or using scented products like deodorant, soaps and laundry detergents. I absolutely avoid cigarette smoke and vehicle exhaust fumes, both of which seem to have the power to throw me into a full-blown relapse. I launder my bedding in hot water with a few drops of eucalyptus oil after reading that it kills dust mites and their eggs. I don't use chemicals to clean my house or to keep up my yard. The list is long and many of these things are quite simple to eliminate.

Toxins are everywhere in this modern world. I figure it's impossible for me to avoid them all. But I found that I can control my exposure in a lot of obvious problem areas. Any little bit of control over this illness is most welcome. I often felt so victimized by the CFS that it felt good to have a strategy to help myself.

Five

Throughout my illness I have struggled with depression. I didn't want to take anti-depressant medication and so really worked at other ways to respond to it. It is quite natural for people living in pain and with the isolation of chronic sickness to feel depressed. Depression isn't always negative, I would reason, something to get rid of or get over. It can be seen instead as healing trying to assert itself. Issues were just knocking at the door. When I opened it I could see many things.

The first was the shame I attached to breaking commitments. This was a source of suffering for me as my health forced me to drop old roles like being sociable, being "there" for my friends, joining the after-work crowd for drinks, keeping our home clean and comfortable. I had to let the shame in. Breath into it. Examine it without judgment.

I saw that I was trying to define myself, or who I thought I should be, based on my pre-illness life. I was feeling drawn back into my old roles for comfort. I was absorbed in my goal to get back where I had been, not considering that where I was in that moment was even slightly okay. I yearned for my lost definitions. It was common to find myself agreeing to do things that had worked before I became ill. The need to re-work my daily patterns and expectations felt monumental, like going through early childhood all over again. I had to try living without definitions for a while and then learn to be flexible around the idea of re-defining myself. I tried to comfort myself by asking, "What in nature is static?"

The fact that we are comforted by definitions that turn around and bite us when we don't live up to them should tell us something about their inherent danger. Stress just ages the body and chronic illness is very stressful, even more so if you keep all these expectations in your life. I saw so many people with CFS trying desperately to hang on to the person and the life they had built. Struggling and resisting. I could see what an art it is be able to live in the moment and to be open to what is there instead of chasing what might be or what once was. I learned that if I had no plans, then not being able to carry plans out was not an issue. A tiny shift in perspective could let me off the hook.

> No plans =
> no aborted plans =
> no reason to be reminded that I can't keep plans because I'm too sick =
> no reason to feel ashamed or that I'd let others down.

It does not have to be forever. It is just for this day. I'll just be spontaneous.

Another source of depression came from my concern over what others thought of me. For some reason I can't quite figure, we give a lot of lip service in our culture to the body-mind connection. But when a person has an illness that can be exacerbated by stress we somehow make that shameful. "Oh," we think to ourselves, "It's all in her head." I sometimes sensed people growing weary of my illness and expecting that I should be able to somehow just snap myself out of it. I've rarely felt such loneliness. If I told them all that I was doing to help myself, all the inner work, all the symptoms and how they impacted me, I would sound like a whiner and a total bore. If I said nothing they thought, "What's the problem?…She doesn't look sick to me."

Then there was the career. That a lot of my sense of self worth was wrapped up in my work came as no surprise. I had no reason to have noticed this before. I guess when there is no conflict, I'm less likely to pay attention to things. So I found myself desperate to make sense of the ocean of new feelings I was experiencing. I knew intellectually that I had intrinsic value but I couldn't get in touch with it any deeper than that. I tried mental exercises. I continued to approach new projects and make commitments that I would ultimately fail to keep. As if I wasn't depressed enough, my start/stop behavior was dragging me further down.

I eventually had to admit to myself that I couldn't do it. All of this trial and error was just compounding my grief and fear. I had to figure out how to just be. I found it very helpful to pay attention to my tendency to see every bad thing as permanent and to remind myself that few things are.

During this time I gleaned a lot about our culture here in North America with regard to illness and personal value. We have television commercials advertising drugs that suppress your awareness of your symptoms so you can go to work sick. It's considered self-indulgent to take more than two days off of work to nurse a cold. We look to the people who come in to work in spite of feeling ill as examples of dedication and loyalty. We call it a "good work ethic." It's no wonder those of us with chronic illness have so much trouble giving ourselves permission to take the time we need to focus on getting well. As a culture, we encourage the opposite.

People with CFS and other chronic, subtle illnesses, face this cultural insensitivity constantly. And just to top it off, our closest loved ones may be skeptical and unable to relate to what we're going through. Doctors often leave us feeling to blame and inferior. The culture tells us we're lazy or self-indulgent. It can be almost unbearable to face the doubt of spouses, family, friends. Before I knew what I was doing, I found that I had taken on the task of convincing everyone that I was really sick. This is certainly not where you should be putting precious energy! Recognizing the absurdity of it helped me to let it go. Fussing over what everyone else might be thinking was poor use of my emotional energy. I just had to trust that those people would come to whatever truth that they could live with. And I would live with mine.

Fear is another mighty companion. When did I become so afraid of being tired? Everytime I got tired, I would go into the fear of a relapse. I had to consciously work to bring this into perspective. I had to work to draw my own attention to the relationship between my tiredness and the fact that I hadn't slept well the night before. Perfectly normal. *I didn't sleep well last night because setting the clocks for daylight savings time threw me off and I was also a bit wired yesterday from a beautiful, sunny weekend.* This became my mantra as I fumbled through the first Monday in April one year. My eyes ached and longed to close. Muscles were stiff, sore and barely able to keep me upright. My breath so quiet, I startled myself with a sigh. My face hot, the rest of me chilled. Noticing cause and effect. Intentionally shifting my perception; my viewpoint.

Continuously pointing to the illness as the cause of all of my discomfort convinces the subconscious and thereby reinforces and strengthens the illness. I was just plain tired. Nothing else.

The illness is real. It did happen to me. It does affect the choices I can make in my life. But convincing myself all the way deep into my subconscious that I am a vicitm of it takes away any sense of personal responsibility and gives me permission to give up. It eventually creates an excuse for me not to take any risks and then I am simply surviving and not really living.

Journal Entry, June 12, 1994:
A real couch Saturday. Very tired and achy and allergy and isolated. Small burst of energy allowed me to do dishes and prepare dinner and grocery shop, though with difficulty. Made two phone calls from the stack of those to do. Read a lot. Napped. Not much appetite. A bit of anxiety and fear about being

too sick to work or have a life. Watching my body and noticing a heaviness to my breath.

This is my second day on a trial of Prozac for depression. I know I tend to be hyper-vigilant on body-talk. My anxiety makes me do it when I try a new medication. Drugs scare me.

I exercised for one minute on the Stairmaster. Truly two minutes would've been pushing it and would keep me off it awhile. I want to try to build back up to twenty minutes but if I push I'll never make it. The CFS book I'm reading says this is how it should be. It says to start with three minutes.

While I wasn't working and was able to focus more on healing myself, I learned to live in a different way. If I tried to live the old way, I would just fail and feel worse. Some of the things I changed included keeping my calendar as empty as possible and considering all appointments tentative; I became more able to let them go easily. I took my time in the morning, evaluating my mood and energy levels before agreeing to any plans. I let the answering machine handle a call if I felt too comfortable to move at the moment the phone rang. I recognized that housework could wait another hour, another day, even another week. I learned to say no in case my illness thrived on being an excuse for my weak self-esteem. And I fought to sort out when no was the simple answer and had nothing to do with being sick.

My progress could be measured in fits and starts, and there was rarely anything linear about it. In time, I saw that it had to be okay to consider my own comfort a priority. I made a list of all of the things that made me comfortable, like feeling warm enough at all times. I saw how often I sat shivering under blankets instead of cranking up the heat a little. I decided that I needed to work on this tendency of mine to ignore my body's needs during this special time.

I usually tried to prepare the evening meal for my family because it made me feel good to do so. Each of us has to choose where we are to put our limited energy stores. When I quit my job it was a way of acknowledging that I didn't have energy to work and to be there for my husband, so I was consciously choosing my marriage as my priority. Preparing dinner was a symbol of this commitment in my mind. Often I did not succeed in this goal, but I tried not to get down on myself about it. If there was any pressure there, my loving gesture might become a chore—increasingly difficult to perform as my anxiety around it escalated on the days I felt too sick to move.

Six

Journal Entry, November 23, 1994:

A useless, immobile, unsociable, sleepy, lethargic day. I hate these days! Hate feeling like such a lump on a log! Feel guilty; fear Keith will think I'm useless and just leave me for someone more fun. I can't believe how immature I'm being. Tomorrow can be completely different, I know. I can't imagine ever having a life again!

Just so tired! Most people have no idea how hard it is for me to get together. I really need to stop care-taking their feelings and learn to say no to all the invitations/expectations.

If Keith was here I wouldn't feel so bad. Poor guy. What a burden I must be depending on him to be my lifeline to the outside world. And what a sport he is. Sometimes I get scared he'll leave. Not that I think he would, but what is scary is that I think it would be reasonable for him to!

Somewhere I heard "Humble tasks are the opportunity to do the ordinary well." I must find the poetry in every action.

I get so stale. The house feels boring. There is no real joy anywhere. I get frustrated with the difficulty of keeping up routines. I just have to grab stuff when I have a good day. I try to exercise lightly Monday/Wednesday/Friday, but just went two weeks with none. I was doing one household chore a day, but stopped that three or so weeks ago. I was trying to garden every morning because it's therapeutic and sweet, but only do it maybe twice a month. Maybe this is another lesson for me—to give up having goals; my need for structure. I'm rather forced to give these up—trying to be a good wife, the dream of adopting a baby, so many things! I can only take things a day at a time for real now. If tomorrow is a good day—I'll do what I can. If it's not—I'll do what I can.

I dream a lot about what my life would be like if I was different.

Some of us get so sick for so long that we can hardly lift our heads off the pillow to say hello. The last thing we need is to feel we need to take care of someone else's needs or feel we have to entertain someone. How many of us are secure

31

enough in our relationships that our minds don't ever wander into wondering just when they'll reach their limit and leave us for greener sights.

Keith, and I had to learn a new way to be in our lives together when I got sick and, particularly, when it looked like things weren't going to be changing anytime too soon. Everything felt noticeably awkward at first, but neither of us acknowledged out loud what was happening. It took some time before we spat it out, tried to come up with a formula we could follow when the idea of activity came up. This was a primary issue for us.

Keith is a sensitive, thoughtful husband whose love endured the strain of CFS admirably. Scenario: a bright and sunny day. I imagine how the parks are full of the city's people cycling, roller blading, pushing baby strollers. On such a day it is only natural that my healthy husband would have an itching to be on the move…get out the old bicycles and pedal around town or walk to Rudolph's, our favorite coffee house, for an espresso.

The first few years of my illness I faced the constant chore of reminding everyone that I was sick. I didn't look sick. My smile was still on my face (of course it was when I was *with* people! I didn't forget how to be kind or polite or lose my love for others!). People who were used to my previous level of activity needed some kind of reminding that things had changed. So I talked about my situation. I explained symptoms. I tried to balance my desire not to be seen as a whiner with the need to keep reminding people that things had changed for me so they would drop the expectations. Flustered, I sometimes got angry at Keith when he would suggest an activity that required—well—moving! It seemed the only way to give people the message that I could no longer do the things I used to be able to do was to constantly complain, and that made me like myself less and kept me more focused on my symptoms than I wanted to be.

Keith developed an understandable hesitancy to suggest we partake in any of the activities we had been accustomed to. He swallowed his fear that I was "giving up" and became quiet about what *he* wanted and what *he* needed and now things were not so good for either of us. It wasn't just that he was afraid that I would get mad at him and think him insensitive. He didn't want me to feel guilty about having to say no to his suggestions if I wasn't feeling well enough. I certainly wasn't the only one struggling to deal with CFS.

In spite of my fear that he might get fed up and leave, I realized that partners don't usually love each other just to have someone to roller skate with. There was an obvious need for some adjustments while I learned to trust that Keith was of the more evolved variety and could love me still, even through this.

Pretty early along, we entered couples counseling to help sort out the negative impact my illness was having on our lives. He did have his share of doubts about my inconsistent symptoms and felt guilty about these. He wasn't ignorant of the controversy surrounding this "yuppie flu" and had his moments of resentment. It was hard for him too. Right or wrong, that just felt like more unfairness and burden on me.

Being a chronically ill person living with a well spouse definitely brought it's share of guilt. I suppose that guilt finds it's way into the lives of everyone with a chronic illness, no matter who one lives with. There's guilt as you drop household responsibilities, guilt as you turn down social invitations, guilt as you are forced to lose your income, and guilt as you put on weight from the inactivity, the hormonal chaos, and the tasty morsels of forbidden foods that are hard to resist when you are able to partake in so few truly pleasurable pursuits.

Guilt is a big issue. I was ever aware of it as I struggled to say no when I had to to all those invitations from well-meaning friends.

If you had a problem saying no before you got sick, CFS is here to teach you how to do it once and for all. Even if you continue to say yes when you mean no (fear, guilt) there will come a time when you understand that this illness is no game or brief visitation. It is here for the long haul and the sooner you learn to adjust your life accordingly the more of a life you will have. I don't believe we do half as much physical harm when we engage in activities we wanted to say no to as we do emotional harm, which then begets the physical. What goes on in the mind is reflected in the health of the body. Stress exacerbates illness. It is the body-mind chemistry at work. So, the self is ignored—at what cost? Who have we given our power to? With no power, how are we to rebuild our lives? It was really, really hard for me to stop worrying about how I was impacting my loved ones. I couldn't just will myself better. I knew I shouldn't feel I failed, but there it was.

Unless you are consistently listless and bedridden with a smogged-in brain, those around you may be confused by the variability of your energy. I always felt like I had some explaining to do if I was seen out and about. Interest in the world around you and unrealistic ambition can be the bane of people with CFS. I also came to value the time that I was alone. It felt like the only time I could be really honest about how bad I felt. Around others, I was much too aware and concerned about what they were thinking or needing from me. I did not want to be perceived as a complainer so I would downplay my discomfort.

I came to see my own guilt as a valuable teacher when I began to look more closely at the high standards and expectations I had of myself. For instance, on a barely conscious level I thought it absolutely imperative to always please others, to never let anyone down and I thought I knew what others wanted of me. I thought that if I let others know how defeated I felt by this illness, they would judge me as weak and any respect I may have earned from them would drop a few notches. I had to learn to respect that I was changed and to trust that others could deal with it. Really, I wasn't displaying much respect for my friends if I believed they were unable to handle me and my illness.

At home it seemed so many critters and people I lived with depended on me in large part for their comfort and sense of well-being. I fed, nurtured, groomed and provided companionship. I was "mom." Letting go of these roles as they had been was extremely difficult and I held on far longer than perhaps was healthy for me.

I've often wondered…if I had just let go of all of these roles and struggles early on, would I have had a much shorter illness? As I moved through my fifth, sixth, seventh year of CFS I would cringe remembering how I pushed myself to keep working when I felt so ill. Working so hard to keep going in a role that didn't suit me any longer may have prolonged a condition that might have abated in a year. I will never know for sure, but research is showing that early diagnosis, treatment and rest does equate with less disability in the long-term.

The need to redefine myself was clear. But none of the definitions that I saw before me had much appeal. If I shook off all the ways I had defined myself in the past, what was left? What role did I truly have the energy for? Who was I here for? *What* was I here for?

I guess a large part of my own difficulty came from my habit of second guessing what others expected of me. How ripped off would Keith feel if I just stopped being the homemaker? How long would he tolerate it? The answer was probably much longer than I could, but I projected my need to feel valuable—and defined value as production or contribution—onto Keith, and was unable to see things any other way.

And guilt, of course, couldn't be satisfied eating away at me alone. It had to have Keith, too. His guilt, like mine, was a confused mass of self-loathing and doubt. He was feeling things that he felt no good man should. His resentment at me for not contributing money, labor, love to the household and relationship seemed cruel to him, but he couldn't deny it.

Someone wisely noted that we think of sick people as either dying or getting better. People with CFS do neither. There is no model for how loved-ones should behave.

Keith, in fact, wanted me well above all else. I did the relationship a disservice by not trusting that my role went deeper than dishwasher/food-preparer and could survive this. More harm may have been done by not taking proper care to ensure the best and speediest recovery for myself, whatever it took.

I was all too aware of the sacrifices Keith had to make during this time. This was not his dream marriage and now years had gone by and it looked like the dream would have to be re-worked. He was aware of my limitations (more so, he claims, than I myself was) and he tiptoed around me fearful of suggesting we do something fun on one of my bad days. We talked about this in circles; a way he could suggest activities he would like to do together while allowing me the freedom to say no without feeling guilty. I had to remember to respect my partner's feelings and needs even as I struggled to face my physical losses and my considerably diminished life. I was definitely limited. I wouldn't be going skydiving. Ever. Not even on my best days. Keith would often comment to me, "I'm not mature enough for this." I appreciated his insight and honesty and felt so blessed to have him as my partner. So many people are facing this illness alone or with partners who cannot come to terms and even leave.

Gradually, Keith and I found a lot of passive activities we could enjoy together. Going to the movies, eating out, renting videos, picnics (we bought prepared stuff at a deli), a soft walk in the evening. We developed some strategies such as "dinner on our own" which was our code when I was too fatigued to prepare dinner and didn't want him to feel responsible for feeding us. Each of us would just be responsible for ourselves. Then I could grab a simple sandwich or heat something for myself in the microwave. Keith would often offer to cook for us both, but being on our own took the pressure off each of us and allowed us to use our energy in other areas. Over time we came to cherish our comforting routine, settling into our middle age with a blanket, some cocoa and a good book.

Seven

Journal Entry, April 8, 1995:
I haven't always looked at CFS as a way to avoid my emotions but, rather, as a
way to put them starkly in-my-face. When I finally quit working and was alone
with myself so much, I remember struggling to be comfortable in the quiet. I
kept trying to fill my life with distractions; projects, school, volunteer work. It
seems that work had been an adequate distraction until it became emotionally
painful itself. Seems like CFS is a wake-up call to look at your emotional pain. In
his book, Healing Back Pain, *Dr. John Sarno suggests that pain or other symp-*
toms can be a distraction from our emotions and that if something else serves
the purpose of distraction or if we process the emotion we will be able to let go
of the pain. I have noticed how symptoms sometimes disappear when my
attention is shifted by a major life event.

As someone who is interested in the topics of psychology and health, I was aware that there could exist the possibility that, on some level, I really didn't want to get well. This sounded so absurd to me, yet I knew enough about the subconscious mind to respect how powerful it is and how utterly unaware we can be. I am not vain enough to consider myself exempt from such a distasteful possibility. I had to fight off my own revulsion at the suggestion that, although I may not have brought this illness on, I could be somehow sustaining it—even subconsciously. Somehow my shame was overruled by my cognizance of this as an innocent condition of human nature. And I can't honestly say that I hadn't noticed that my illness could be used as a kind of permission slip to get out of unpleasant things. I vowed to spend some serious time examining the concept from every angle. I really had to know. I'd do whatever it took to get well.

I wanted to look closely and see if there was some kind of pay-off for being sick that might be sub-consciously keeping me stuck. A term I've heard used in connection with chronic conditions is "secondary gain." This refers to any way in which the person with chronic illness might stand to *gain* from being sick to a degree that he or she consciously or unconsciously doesn't want to give up the illness. It sounds so offensive, like the party line that you create your own illness and therefore you can make yourself well. In fact, I have heard that the term is used primarily by insurance companies to delay or deny benefits. In spite of the negative connotation, I think it's a valuable question to ask ourselves if we can shed the defensiveness caused by repeated experiences we've had with it's-all-in-your-head thinking. Surely this line of questioning can make us feel vulnerable, and the level of honesty and self-awareness required for answers can be difficult. But I felt nagged by it. I needed to answer it for myself.

I found it immediately helpful to read the book I referred to in the previous Journal Entry, *Healing Back Pain, The Mind-Body Connection*, by Dr. John E. Sarno (1991). A friend of mine who also struggled with chronic illness pointed this book out to me when she experienced an enormous shift in her recovery after reading it. Dr. Sarno's research shows that the idea of secondary gain presupposes a structural explanation for the pain, making it likely that you will work on changing the structure rather than the emotion that belies it. He cites that pain and some illnesses are often preceeded by emotion, yet consistently we appoach it by looking for a structural cause or injury and treating that while ignoring the very real underlying emotional roots. It's like mopping up the floor of a flooded room while leaving the faucet running and the sink overflowing. His point is that it's the emotions that need our attention.

If I am to be honest, I will have to admit that I noticed that my symptoms would worsen when I would think seriously about returning to work. I had always turned away from any deep investigating of this phenomenon, since it smacked of me being responsible for creating or at least sustaining my illness. But in the shadows of my consciousness I silently nodded, acknowledging the problems I had with assertiveness at work. Bullies always seemed to find me and I was unable to say no to nice people. I felt too vulnerable.

Accordingly, I decided to look deeply into the questions about pay-off, while monitoring my explorations to be sure I included any emotional story that may be behind them. I began by considering the question of being sick to gain good old-fashioned attention and then rejected that almost instantly. For one thing, I had no shortage of positive attention prior to becomming ill that would have made me seek the negative. I had many people in my life who had *always* fussed and given me ample attention. And most people didn't realize how seriously ill I was because they didn't actually see it. Also, my career was my arena, if you will, and it was there that I got the most attention. But the illness forced me out of that career. I lost every description I held of myself along with the entire feedback system that kept my confidence up. I had been active and creative in my work, and had the respect of people I respected. For me, work had been a sublime vehicle for gaining any attention I might crave. So, the idea of gaining attention at least, didn't seem to fit.

Perhaps ironically, another potential pay-off could have been getting to leave my job. Here I see a hint of truth in that my job, at the time that I left it, had become significantly stressful. Not liking confrontation, I had a difficult time remaining assertive and confident when situations called me to be.

A significant thing that bothered me at work was that I had begun noticing that I wasn't always thinking clearly enough to perform my job at the level others depended on. In my line of work with adults with developmental disabilities, lives were often literally shaped by my decisions, usually as part of a team, but sometimes individually. This was a great responsibility. If someone needed a particular service or creative solution such as an assistive device or technology to help them function in their daily lives, I usually knew where they could get it and how to get it for them. But lately I had found myself missing obvious solutions when a colleague would suggest something that should have been the first thing that came to my mind, but didn't. This was happening with more and more frequency. My brain didn't seem to be fully engaging in what I was doing, saying or even thinking, something that I later learned was a hallmark symptom of CFS.

I felt a great sense of responsibility towards the people I had chosen to serve in my work. These people depended on others to a large degree to make decisions for them that had great impact on their futures. Many people working with the developmentally disabled population seem to be there because it's the only place they can find themselves powerful and dominant, and they often seemed to make sweeping decisions with hardly a care for the client. Sometimes I envied their ability to do this work and sleep so easily at night after ordering psychotropic drugs for someone or deciding a client wouldn't be able to handle an opportunity that had presented itself—one that might have greatly enhanced his or her life. I was very serious about my work and needed a clear, working mind to do my job well.

During the several months preceeding my resignation there was also a lot of political turmoil at work that directly impacted me. This bothered me a great deal because I loved the job itself. I loved what I did. I had dedicated seventeen years of my life to promoting a paradigm shift in the prevailing public belief system that hindered the lives of a certain segment of the population. I enjoyed my successes, however small. This job carried a huge emotional component in that I cared immensely about the people I chose to serve. Many social service jobs have that emotional aspect; you have to care to be effective.

I will concede that the dysfunction and turmoil at work was uncomfortable for me, but to dump my career over a single period of upheaval seems a bit of an overreaction, don't you think? What is more likely, and what my counselor and doctor had been telling me, is that the stress in this job *exacerbated* my symptoms, sending me over the precipice where my ability to function departed, and I was forced to quit.

Continuing my line of self-questioning, I looked at another aspect of my career that I wanted to explore: the level of responsibility I had held. I can remember feeling uncomfortable, even overwhelmed at times with the responsibility I had been given over other people's lives. In my experience, this power sometimes seems to be given out rather recklessly in social services. I suffered at times from the "imposter phenomenon," having earned my stripes through experience alone in a culture where formal education is valued more. Sometimes I would become suddenly panicked as I looked upon the myriad of tasks I was juggling. I can see how, at these times, I wanted out. It's hard to explain this, but it was like being afraid that I would "lose it" and mess everything up. It made sense to me that the sicker I got, the more frequent these feelings became; because the sicker I got, the harder it was for me to maintain my normal pace. It became cognitively difficult for me to keep track of it all. The responsibility weighed on me at those times. I could see myself now, considering returning to work when I recovered, yet panicked at the thought of resuming that same career. Because by now I was feeling less competent. I knew I didn't want to re-create that scenario again in my life. I didn't like it.

The flip side of not having to work is getting to stay home. Now, this may sound beautiful to many people. I admit that I wished for that kind of life many times while working—pre-illness. But my stay-at-home dream looked nothing like the reality I got. In my dreams I was healthy at home, volunteering here and there, cooking gourmet meals, taking classes, meditating regularly, having babies and then raising them with calm wisdom. This is not what I got. I got day after day of being able to do no more than lie on the couch. Instead of homemade vegetarian meals, I got fast food and had to postpone motherhood permanently, as it would turn out—easily the biggest disappointment of my life. Talk shows became my window to the outside world, a sort of substitution for the real interactions with others I was missing. My brain was motivated to have the dream but my body was in no way cooperating. Boredom became a frequent visitor. The highlight of my day was an afternoon cup of flavored coffee with a cookie. *Not* the stay-at-home picture I would wish for, so if this was to be my pay-off you would think my illness would have scampered out of there with its tail between its legs once it found out that a leisurely bliss was not to be had. Failed, its job would've been finished.

Receiving disability benefits that were one fourth of the professional salary I had been earning also did not feel like any kind of pay-off that might invest me in remaining ill. It did ease my fears regarding our financial well-being while I was not bringing home a paycheck, but I was so motivated to get back to working that I was not at all seduced by the "easy money," nor was it enough to sustain a lavish, stay-at-home lifestyle. I do know people who have propped themselves up with so many marvelous social services and benefits that I wonder how they will ever "allow" themselves to recover and lose all of it. It might be difficult on a sub-conscious level to allow yourself to get better if it means you will have to forfeit a monthly Social Security check, free housekeeping, reduced rent if you live in sub-sidized housing, free school/re-training, free groceries, and handicapped parking access—not to mention all the time and effort you had to spend convincing everyone you were sick enough to get these benefits. Because most of these ser-vices operate on an 'all or nothing' level, you lose them once you recover your ability to work—even if you cannot manage a full-time job or to return to a field where it is at all possible to earn enough money to live.

As I continued to parade the contents of my life before me, looking for any real gain to staying sick, I was in touch with a sense of relief to let go of much of my old life. But what was left was a chunk of empty, painful time that was most unpredictable and uncomfortable for a person whose ambition and motivation remained consistently intact. I experienced a lot of restlessness and frustration because I couldn't think of anything that I was capable of doing in my current condition. I desperately looked for a way to define myself through tasks and repeatedly fought my own internalized beliefs about personal value. I couldn't seem to stop searching for stuff to fill my time.

I knew I needed to stay with this empty space in spite of my discomfort with inactivity. Still, the body-mind connection is well documented and I wanted to examine myself closely and honestly so that I could be assured that I wasn't miss-ing something that was literally *making me sick*. I had given it a good effort and eventually became satisfied that I gained little and, in fact, lost much by becom-ing ill. So I turned my thoughts to any potential pay-offs for *staying* sick. Were there any surprise gains? Built-in scapegoats? Were any of the positives that had resulted from these forced changes so awesomely wonderful and dependent on my illness that I couldn't let go of them?

Like many of us, I often ignore or try to hide from my uncomfortable feelings. But I believe that my progress towards "healing" came from practicing just *being with* these feelings. CFS forces this somewhat. Too ill to move, there isn't much we can do to run and hide. We are a captive audience to our internal process. I found that taking the time to observe my resistances and frustrations in a non-judgmental fashion could actually soften them. It is necessary work to make this kind of peace with your own grieving for your lost life. Healing is found some-where between resistance and resignation.

I began taking a close look at my new life and how I had re-arranged myself and everything around me. I was gradually learning to live empty of expectations and had begun to understand and to care enough about myself to want to be good to me. Each activity in which I participated was a gift to myself, in that I had examined it for benefit or potential harmful side effects prior to allowing it into my life.

In some ways I could see that I had grown to actually like my life. I could be filled with joy sitting quietly on the veranda watching the birds pick sunflower seeds from the pebbly ground around the feeder. I had better energy because I wasn't constantly over-doing, and I kept moderate exercise in my life after trial-and-error learning taught me how much better it made me feel. I found good nutrition that was right for *me* (which is to say not necessarily textbook right) and I followed it faithfully, having noticed an improvement in my stamina and mood. In time, I was able to loosen up some of these strategies, but they served me well as a pathway out of the acute phase of my CFS. I had begun to volunteer from my home for an animal welfare organization, calling pet owners to check on their animals after surgeries and fostering abandoned kittens until they were placed in good homes. This was important to me; it fed my soul yet required little of me in terms of energy. Most importantly I could do it in my pj's and a house full of kit-tens is great for lifting the spirits!

It took years for me to get to this point. I tried to keep just this much and no more in my life and it worked well for me. I feared losing my disability benefits and being flung back into the workplace where *my* needs would come last. I feared doing anything out of necessity and falling so far backwards into sickness that I would be forced to let go of everything I'd gained.

Yes, in this there could be some gain in remaining sick, except that my moti-vation to work was intact. I still wanted to contribute, to participate in life. My dream for the future included working again, but in a way that was healthy and that nourished me. For me, it couldn't be about money. It was just about partici-pating and living my life in a soulful way. I had gradually managed to turn every-thing around so that most things that entered my life were good for me. As my health continued to improve, I knew it would be challenging to remember all of this.

Having identified a lack of assertiveness and a tendency to feel overwhelmed as possible 'reasons' to take shelter in sickness, I could see that part of my work was to learn to be careful and to say 'no' when that is what I meant. I was unwilling to assume anything when it came to my subconscious mind and vowed to live with more courage.

Looking inward for bits of truth about any role my subconscious might be playing in my illness produced a gift of clarity that fostered a shift in my thinking. That shift led to a peace with myself I had never known before. I felt certain that I wasn't holding myself back. Because I had spent this time of honest reflection, I would not have to live with suspicion that I was being weak or selfish or a nut case! My body and mind were at last in partnership, on a journey together, our knapsacks full of dedication and commitment to a continuous sorting through the stuff of life, filtering out what, for me was poisonous and letting in things of brightness, warmth, nurture, purity.

And so it came to pass that we moved to Seattle for Keith to pursue his dream of going to art school, given that I had at least temporarily been forced to relinquish any such sky-blue dreams of my own. The forced solitude of life in a place where we knew only a couple of people initially turned out to be a blessing. I was able to rest more and was relieved from all of those social obligations to which I could never say 'no.' What better way to be with my questions, watching squirrels scamper in my own yard, the telephone quiet, the only voices from the wind, the critters, and my own heart.

Eight

Journal Entry November 22, 1995:

I always have to have a good reason to take a nap or to stay home. Today I took a nap not because I have CFS but because I simply wanted to.

Journal Entry January December 15, 1995:

I resist accepting that this is all there is to me; that this is all there is to my life.

Journal Entry January 28, 1996:

I've noticed that although I still have relapses, my remissions are more fully healthy, convincing me that I am getting better overall. Even though I just had a month-long relapse, it followed a very healthy course such as the one I've just entered.

I also notice a lot of anxiety and uncomfortable, urgency-laden, obsessive thinking goes on during my relapses. Part of this may be the depression of the relapse, but I notice it tends to culminate in the ultimate solution to whatever it is I'm perseverating about. So, it seems to be a stewing sort of healing that may be necessary in some way. Sort of an incubation period preceding a personal insight. Seems I have to struggle for personal insights while insights into other people's situations come quite easily. I'm convinced that emotional healing will lead to physical healing.

I am sitting on the floor in one of the bedrooms of our house. There is a sliding glass door right in front of me. I just completed some yoga postures. A squirrel came by and looked at me closely through the glass. Now a great orange cat is ambushing the birds. This window is like a giant diorama. It is misty outside.

I took to stretching with yoga each morning after my shower. The warm water of the shower seems to help prepare my muscles for relaxing and stretching. I do about five postures sitting, five lying supine, and about five standing. Kneeling and lying prone are too painful for me.

I usually like to follow this with a sitting meditation. My body cannot sit in one posture for long, though I believe the yoga helps, so I have modified it such that it's divided into three segments. The important thing is to be able to let go of rigid standards like, "If I can't sit absolutely still for twenty minutes I can't meditate." I sit quietly for as long as I tolerate it. Then I lean forward in a stretch; it feels so good. I take a deep breath before I stretch and let it out as I move forward. I hold this position as long as it feels good. I may say an affirmation or visualize something positive for that day while I'm here.

When I perform rituals like this I feel that I am honoring my body and its needs during this illness. Where would I have squeezed this into a working day? I am grateful to have this chance.

At some point I learned, often painfully and definitely slowly, how to take care of myself with CFS without giving over my whole life to it. I learned to listen and to accept my energy level and yet I also learned to challenge myself not to have rigid expectations about my limitations. I couldn't hear myself before. Maybe there had been too much white noise in an attempt to avoid confronting what I might find in my deepest parts. I figured out how to pace my activities, to say no when I needed to, to check in with my body before taking on any activity, and to make activities that helped to heal me my first priority. Shaving my legs is not so important; a regular sleep schedule is.

I learned a lot of this in my career as a teacher. Shoe-tying is a difficult thing to teach someone with intellectual challenges and/or visual or fine motor problems. Rather than frustrate both the learner and myself, I saw that tying a bow had little use in the larger picture of life. One could certainly live nicely without that particular skill. There was, after all, the penny loafer. So, shoe-tying was out; slip-ons were in. CFS asks that we examine our activities in a similar manner. Where are we making more work for ourselves than necessary?

Journal Entry, January 18, 1996:

It's a gray day and I sing in the beauty of fall in the Pacific Northwest. I am on my way home from swimming at the gym and I feel good. There is a great wind blowing, filling the leaves that have fallen from the trees with an urge to dance in circles five feet off the ground. I indulge in the excitement inherent in the changing of the seasons.

Just yesterday I stared out the picture window in my living room. The day was dark and rain threatened, leaking sprinkles now and then. I sighed in deep waves of depression. Doom and gloom. My symptoms were severe and I ached from one end to the other. I couldn't see myself feeling any different, not in the past, or the future.

And so it goes with CFS. There is this constant in and out, home and not-home, joy and grief. A person must learn to be OKAY with the changing and shifting of body and mood. It may change at any hour, or from one day to the next, one week to the next or even one year to the next. The weather is virtually the same weather, you are in the same relationships, you weigh the same, yet the color drains and then paints itself back into the picture of your life with no logic or pattern. It can be most disconcerting indeed!

I try to be a positive person. I'd like to think that I have mostly faced this illness with courage and grace. But these down days have the power to wipe out every good thought I ever had. The memory of another self becomes illusive. Life looks like a procession of dark days. Too sick to go outside. Chilled from the inside out. Too buried in mental fog to pull an insight out of its gift-wrap. I question all of my dreams and ambitions, those I discover on the good days. How can I possibly do or be anything but this sick, sorry mess!

Seems I have to reinvent myself every day. It becomes so tiring and feels so useless when yesterday's definition doesn't fit today, doesn't fit tomorrow and on and on.

On the rare good day I feel strong and confident. I am thoughtful and do delightful things for friends and loved ones. I whoosh through the sky on a swing of joy and gratefulness. I am positive and full of life.

Then comes the so-so day. Here I am not so full of life. I may not whoosh through anything, but I'm OKAY and I manage to get dinner on the table with a smile.

And then the bad days come, where I am only full of **it. I am a bore and a complainer, irritable and useless and hard to get along with.

I know I should wise up to the fact that all of this will pass. A bad day will eventually turn back into a good one. It always does. It's such a struggle to trust that bad days would not go on and on indefinitely, and to hope that the good days would likewise stay. Perspective. I know this can save me. But it slips from me over and over again.

When I have finally learned to accept that it is enough to be doing the best I can with what I have on each and every day, I will be freed. How nice to think that my sense of self worth would stay relatively intact no matter what the rest of my insides do.

Sounds so easy. Maybe it is easy. I can believe I am doing the best that I can. Heck! I can even feel a little pride that I have choreographed a rather delicate waltz with such a clumsy partner as CFS. (I must make it look easy, after all, I hear over and over how well I look.)

When I wake up tomorrow morning I will invite myself to dance and I will know that the music and the timing and my steps are the absolute best they can be with whichever partner I find facing me. Yes, sometimes I will dance with Cinderella and some days with Peter Pan. Eyeore may drag my feet one minute and the next I may find myself facing the Devil himself and still I will trust my inner rhythm. Some days I will dance with clouds and some with the rays of the sun. I will dance the taps of little tears and whirl in a great wind five feet off the ground.

Surprisingly, we learned that the weather in this part of the Pacific Northwest was not nearly as damp and dreary as its reputation foretold. In fact, the physical beauty of the area fed my spirit a true chicken soup as I sat on our back porch in eighty-degree sunshine and watched chickadees at the birdfeeder against the backdrop of rhododendron in bloom.

In this quiet frame of mind, I would walk through Seattle's numerous forests, parks and waterways redefining my life and myself. I could feel the shifting that was to mark the beginning of my return to health—one of several steps out of the darkness. I could call this, "the power of joy," and I found it through nature in all of its manifestations. Trees, puppies, squirrels, sunshine sparkling over lakes and Puget Sound. Snow-capped mountain ranges, ferns, bald eagles flying overhead in the city, paths strewn with pine needles, the quiet stillness of morning fog. And this is where I live! The awe seemed to work on some metabolic level, helping my immune system pull itself up out of the murky darkness.

I have felt so thrilled to notice the healing power joy has had on my life. I often make lists of things that please me and then evaluate the degree that they are present in my life. Many things that would be simple enough to incorporate are not getting any attention. It is such a lesson to see on paper what gives us joy and then to ask ourselves what role we are giving them. Many of the items and activities on my list were given no priority or had very little presence in my life. Usually—and not surprisingly—they seemed to slip away at the same times that my depression would be gaining a foothold.

In spite of my progress, my relapses could still throw me into despair. Our new home, far from family and life-long friends, became a mixed blessing as loneliness took over. It was difficult to make new friends since I didn't really make plans and rarely showed up when I would leave anything to spontaneity. I had met other people living with chronic illness and they could understand totally, but I wanted healthy friends too. I needed the humor, the model, to witness the ease. I missed my hometown and longed to see the face of a loved one.

CFS may be a virus, or an immune system dysfunction, or a whatever. Still, there is much of CFS that we can control; things that we unwittingly may "add on" to it. Things like fear can trigger a chemical reaction in the body that can bring pain—never underestimate that biochemistry! We can become lethargic from too little activity, can get depressed when we impose limits on ourselves or stop trying to do the things we love. Our beliefs are very powerful in determining our reality. I don't mean to make any of this sound easy or to trivialize anyone's experience, but I do feel that it is absolutely crucial to recognize that we have some power to improve our situation. It may not be smooth and consistent, but it can relieve so much of our suffering.

If you learn, for instance, of a traumatic childhood event that occurred in December, you may think to yourself that it explains why the holidays have always been so hard for you. Any good holidays you may have had may then be rejected by your memory because they no longer fit your belief about the season. It becomes likely that future holidays will be hard for you because you expect them to be.

One day I was expecting an exterminator to spray my home for carpenter ants. As it turned out, he did not spray that day. Later that evening, I had a resurgence of fatigue and aches. Had the exterminator sprayed as planned, I know I would have attributed my discomfort to the toxic chemicals he'd used to treat the ants in my house. I would have thereafter believed myself to be "sensitive" to that chemical, likely would have generalized it to include other things and I would have altered my life accordingly. From that day forward I might have lived in fear of all chemicals—all because I had misapplied cause and effect in that one situation. This clearly showed me how I might add things to my illness that weren't really there.

I think symptoms can work like this too. It's good to be watchful and to *really* listen to the things you say to yourself.

Nine

I find this excerpt from Stephen Levine's book, *Who Dies?*, most valuable:

> *"I have seen situations where two people of the same age and similar backgrounds had the same pathology and prognosis. One fought his disease using methods that marshaled his aggression to combat the illness that encouraged him to think of himself as a victim, to regard illness as an unnatural intrusion. He became tighter and more frightened, grasping at life. In days of lessening symptoms he felt quite "up" and "wonderful." In moments of noticeable illness, he felt "down" and "awful." One could see how his self-value was predicated on how well he was able to heal himself. When symptoms asserted themselves his feeling of value diminished and the aggression he was cultivating turned inward in self-loathing and guilt.*
>
> *"The other fellow recognized the disease as a message of work to be done. He strove to come back into harmony, to bring the heart and mind into balance, to improve the quality of his life while harmonizing what seemed out of kilter. Rather than putting his energy into only extending life he went deeper into the richness that made life worth living. He did not hold shallow, 'hanging tough' as the other fellow put it."*

In my middle age, I slowly awakened to an awareness of an incapacitating aspect of CFS that I had never considered. A new kind of despair had taken hold of me over a long period of time. Being a thinker, I journaled and pondered through walks in the woods, never putting my finger directly on it, seeing the symptoms, but not the cause. Then one morning I had the big *aha* and understood. Happy to have something to work with (in *my* mind, understanding is the road to solution), yet sad to see more evidence of my profound, ongoing relationship with this syndrome. I felt like I had discovered a chapter left unwritten in all the literature I had consumed. CFS in middle age. CFS as it settles itself into a comfortable *lifetime* inside the human body. How it makes itself at home, claims a favorite chair in the living room and then doesn't want to budge from it's spot.

After living for more than a decade with CFS, I felt I had adapted fairly well. As long as I held to a routine and a pace that it took me the first five years to figure out—my CFS zone—I seemed to have a decent life that wasn't constantly referenced and dictated by my illness. The routine and pace had become so natural for me that it didn't take any effort or thought, I simply considered it my life-style.

We all know about comfort zones. They are like boxes we create around our selves and our lives where we remain comfortable as long as we don't attempt to do anything outside the box. As I got older, I found them to be even more stub-born and harder to break free of: watching *The X Files* on Sunday nights, reading in bed from 10–11pm, lengthy periods of solitude and silence. These made up the rhythm of my daily existence and although, on the one hand, I resisted mak-ing any claims about their hold on me, I gradually grew to cling to them like a babe to its mother. You know how good it feels to fall into bed at the end of a long, busy day? That's how my routine felt—like falling into bed.

I found myself incredibly lonely for companionship, yet was puzzled by my inertia in doing anything about it. Flying home to see my much beloved and incredibly missed family and friends had turned into a dozen obstacles: the need to get up early for the flight, the exhaustion from non-stop visiting and activity, working through the anxiety around flying itself, anticipating the necessary recovery time when I would arrive and again on returning home, and therefore being able to take a significant chunk of time away, the expense (if I wanted some solitude and a chance to refresh) of a hotel, the cost of the flight since I panic driving on the freeway and therefore needed to take two flights to get home at twice the expense, missing my husband and pets and my sweet routine. I would become overwhelmed trying to make my plans. This was simply impossible for me to reconcile with my intense desire to be with loved ones back in California. But this sort of paralysis would always come when my safe routine felt threat-ened. It is undoubtably rooted in my PTSD, which causes me to be easily over-whelmed by fear.

I turned down virtually all social invitations and avoided people if contact included the possibility (obligation?) of making plans. Healthy people just don't understand what making plans feels like to someone with CFS. I didn't want to struggle with feeling judged and misunderstood. I had given up explaining. I could find few souls who could relate—all of them living with chronic illness, more specifically post-polio syndrome, multiple sclerosis, lupus or CFS/FMS.

Another ongoing frustration had become my desire to be involved in charity or volunteer work, yet I couldn't seem to settle on a cause or make a solid com-mitment. I knew from experience that helping others made me feel good. As long as I wasn't doing anything on a regular basis that would qualify as charity work, I bothered myself continuously about the need to do so. I had trouble understand-ing what the hold-up was. Was I merely pressuring myself out of Catholic-girl guilt? Did I think I was worthless unless I gave? Was I plain lazy? Selfish? Or was it just the CFS and my denial of its impact that kept me in this struggle? Perhaps it was as simple as that the CFS left nothing of me to give.

I thought perhaps I wanted too many things at once—close friendships, volunteering, returning to school, taking yoga classes and establishing a regular practice, taking up art or poetry. Maybe this was too much for someone with CFS and I needed to take it one thing at a time. But even when I decided to zero in on one thing I found months passing by and nothing happening. 'What is this inertia?', I asked myself. *Aha*. Not inertia. Comfort with a capital "C" and a stubborn clinging.

It was then that I realized that my CFS routine had become enmeshed with my natural comfort zone and I saw how dependent I had become on it. I am not unfamiliar with the impact of the human comfort zone. It is powerful stuff and we all have the tendency to carve out our little zones as we age. Whenever I investigated or considered expanding the boundaries of my own zone, I felt anxiety and panic. Any time I would try to pull myself out of my solitude I would have a fear reaction. It is reasonable to expect that my anxiety might be related to a fear of having a relapse, but I intuitively knew that more than this was at play.

So easy to nap in the cocoony comfort of our homes in the winter. So lovely to shed expectation. Such a relief to be able to count on sameness, to always know what's next, to live in uncomplicated rhythm. This, at the very least, makes the discomfort of CFS a little more bearable.

It is not at all surprising that isolation takes on the dichotomy of friend/enemy for people living with a chronic illness. The need for rest, the incredible yet unexpected energy it takes simply to carry on a conversation, the difficulty finding people who can understand what your life is like and the consequent judgment from people you hold dear who do not understand, the exhaustion and relapse that often follows attempts to be social. You pull back and become lonely—home alone listening to Joni Mitchell and Enya.

The comfort zone is what we create to cope with our lives. The CFS zone is what I created to cope with my illness. Sometimes we need to break out of our comfort zones to feel alive. I know that these zones, while offering the illusion of safety and control, can in reality be dead zones for me. It made sense to me to respond by trying to break out of the confines in baby steps; to do one small thing a day, or a week, that got me out of the zone, the sameness, and reminded me that I'm a part of this life. I am alive!

Ten

In 1988 I took a turn in the road on my journey through life. I didn't notice any signpost at the time, but I know that it must have been there. The sign would have read: "Chronic Illness Ahead." I didn't see it coming. Perhaps someone had turned the boards around so the arrows were pointing in the wrong directions. Or a shrub had sent its branches reaching to cover the warning. I know it must have been there. I know it. Somehow I just didn't see it until it was too late.

Now as I look around me, I find I am on a new road. I can look back and see where I've been and many things are clear now that were hidden by twists and turns and caves of denial. I am certain that the road ahead is full of still more of the same, but now I have learned this wonderful secret.

I have learned to see that there are hidden gems along the road. I can pick them up. Turn them in my hand. Look at them from the bottom up or the up bottom. I can lick them, smell them, try to throw them and see what happens. One thing I can count on is that they are there. Each time I sit pondering one, I find the path lies smoother before me than it did when I first sat down. Behind me the road has straightened so that I can see where I've been, and looking ahead it's sweeter, simpler, more mine. The trick is in keeping my mind open to the uniqueness of each thing I examine and not assigning it the characteristics of the one I previously held.

This is all about healing and the fortune that I found along the way. It is about truly seeing what lies at my feet. It is awesomely simple and privately brilliant and each of us has a path unique. But I believe the gist of the message is universal. I believe the messenger is the inner self and the message imperative. The Mighty Oz is you.

About eight years into my illness, I suddenly found myself feeling more well than I'd come to expect. What happened? Once my improved health had gotten my attention, things became clear at a rapid pace. It was like I had suddenly found all the gems piled at my feet. I began to find relief as I discovered the soft beauty in letting go of my resistance. The opera of my spiritual self soared and led me to see that I am the conductor. I hold the wand. I write the music. And it can be beautiful.

One of the truths I found at the horizon of my illness was that if I suspended all beliefs I had about the illness itself and how it affected me, many of them were no longer operating as truths. For example, I had learned that sticking to a set sleep schedule was important to my body. I came to believe that if I got up early I would be full of symptoms all of that day. Every time. Of course, once I'd learned this I didn't get up early anymore. So how was I to know that it was no longer true?

I stopped taking sleeping aids and found that I was able to sleep without them. I worked at letting go of thinking twenty four hours a day of my chronic fatigue, which had become such a backdrop to my life. I saw the irony here: at one time it was necessary for me to learn to think of nothing but myself and my immediate needs in order to get well; now I needed to let that go—to undo the done as I found myself more and more well and ready to invite life back in. In my search to define myself I'd picked up another definition—that I am a sick person. It informed my life. It was time to let it go.

I gave away all of my CFS books to a support group. I let subscriptions to CFS and other medical journals lapse. I gave up talking ceaselessly to myself and others about my symptoms. Since all of my behavior had been based on the fact that I was always sick, my continuing belief in that had effectively shut the door on any hope of escape. I had literally left no room for the possibility of recovery. I had been buried in fear, self-pity and resignation. I had become a walking, talking illness. It really was the predominant thing I had thought about. Every day. For eight years. So I dropped it like taking off a pair of shoes after finding you have stepped in dog doo.

I know that my personal biology reacts better to some things than to others and I am always careful to give equal time to the mind and to be alert to the danger of giving this illness power by scripting it too closely. I really feel that my expectations and beliefs can easily override my body's natural state. It is a very fine line. There is my body. There is my mind. Separate and yet not separate, for what one does impacts how I experience the other. I learned to be cautious not to have too many expectations related to my CFS.

I witness this phenomenon frequently living in the Seattle area. The weather is always grist for the conversational mill around here. People are used to commiserating over the rain. My first year here I was surprised to find so many people complaining that it was, "always raining" in Seattle. In the middle of a gorgeous summer with high temperatures and ample sunshine we got a day of light sprinkling. I was astounded to hear many people complaining about how it "always rains in Seattle." When I pointed out the long stretch of sunny days we had just enjoyed, they would argue that it had actually rained more often than I was remembering. The habit, beliefs and expectations of these people did not allow them to fully appreciate that beautiful weather.

Once I had learned to suspend and challenge my many beliefs about my CFS, I was able to notice that my symptoms often abated during the summer months. It is noted in the research literature that many people seem to have a seasonal component to their CFS. Usually the colder weather found me wrapped in a blanket with fever, aches, and chills; very flu-feely.

That first winter with no chills and flu-aches I knew something had shifted in me. I then got through another winter and and observed that the flare-ups of flu-like symptoms came only rarely, were brief, and could be explained by some physical or emotional stressor that was particularly strong at that exact time.

I began to wonder if I might be well. I spent most days in what felt like a good remission, but was it remission or cure? My main symptom at that point was tiredness. Plain old garden variety tired. I also had no stamina, no zip. During the course of my illness I had gone from thirty-five to forty-two years old. What is a healthy forty-two year-old supposed to feel like, I wondered?

In the course of this self-examination, I learned that I had formed hundreds of beliefs about myself in relation to my CFS during the invasion of this illness. These beliefs had caused me to alter my behavior which meant I was giving them lots of power. Learning to challenge them took some practice because they had become so automatic for me.

What I began to see came as a shock. Was the CFS gone? Had it left? When did it go? How long had I been this well? Was I all the way well? How do you tell when a remission is permanent? I was so used to having my hopes dashed by a relapse that I moved along very cautiously.

In time, I came to see that it was not that simple. This was the recovery of *life*, if not complete health. Indeed, the mysteries of human biology and psychology seem always to evade our full understanding. I do see that the things I learned and did to help to heal myself had a very big impact on my experience of CFS and my ability to feel happy and content. I truly had reclaimed my life and embraced the Mighty Wizard—my own mind and heart, my power and my connection—not outside myself, all right here.

I continue to need to click my heels together at times, to remind myself of all that I have learned. To remember, most of all, to notice the vibrant colors of fall as trees holler out their joy and magnificence. To feel the contentment of a warmly lit night, fat socks on my feet, and my dogs and husband nearby. To screw up my eyes and lose myself in the sparkle of faeries playing on water in the sunlight. And to keep believing that, in life, we can either try to expose the magicians tricks and illusions, or just enjoy a world where anything is possible and magic is within the reach of any one of us.

Journal Entry, May 21, 1996:

- *I rarely ache and chill. Truly, when it happens, I can see that I've been stressed, so I rest it away. I'd say it's happened on average one brief time every two or three months over the past year and a half.*

- *I stopped the Elavil and my sleep problems didn't get worse.*

- *If I get up early, I don't pay.*

- *I can do average activity, even exercise (but no aerobics) and not pay.*

- *I don't hurt anywhere. Ever.*

- *I stopped the anti-depressant without event.*

- *My temperature is often normal.*

I still get frequent, brief headaches. It still takes me 1–2 hours to fall asleep. I get confused sometimes. I am often sleepy in the daytime. I really never have any zing. But I think of these as residue. In time they too may decrease or vanish. I think of myself as vulnerable still, like I should be careful not to overdo. I take lots of breaks and have many peaceful, passive pursuits. I'm careful to say no when I mean it.

Journal Entry, June 17, 1996:

Slight relapse lately: achy, symptoms coming in the evenings. Sometimes my glands are tender and I am chilled. In August, we moved to a new neighborhood. In September, I went through major surgery and the weather dropped into fall.

Still no sign of serious symptoms, though. Good energy in the daytime. I'm tolerating a lot of exercise—like a steep five-mile hike up to Wallace Falls. I'm thinking it's time to try part-time work. Something easy, but not boring.

Journal Entry, November 2, 1996:

Got hired for a temporary (four month) job today. Spooky about my stamina. There will be an early morning walk to the bus in the winter chill and dark on my way home = not so thrilling. But I'm ready to challenge the thought that I can't do it. It's a nice office job in a beautiful building with nice people; it's only four days a week and it's temporary—I must remember this. Just a trial to see if I'm able to handle working. I have no idea how I'm going to keep up with all the other stuff of life, but I'll do my best. I can always quit if it doesn't work.

Journal Entry, November 3, 1996:

Off and on freaking over having accepted the job. I guess it's expected after two and a half years on disability. I get scared. I do have good stamina lately and I've given it a long time to settle in. Still I can hardly believe it's real. For so long now I talk to friends about things I'm planning, but never actually do them. I've gotten used to this pretend life and have come to expect that all of my talk is just that. I come alive in the fantasy, but find safety in the hidden knowledge that I'll never actually do it. I've been well enough to fantasize an interesting life. But to really live one?

Journal Entry, November 9, 1996:

Four full days of work and I survived with no CFS symptoms! Yippee!

Journal Entry, November 11, 1996:

CFS symptoms tonight. Mellow, but there. Did lots today, but maybe should have rested more.

Journal Entry, November 12, 1996:

Realized today that I don't need to do it all. I can let up on housework and stuff until I adjust to working. I have to keep hold of the things I've learned about wellness. I can't let old workaholic patterns return...keep my perspective...don't let work claim all of me...it isn't urgent...it isn't the most important thing. Maybe it's because work is where we feel so judged that we get hooked. I have to keep my priorities straight.

CFS LEGACY

I claim good health
I claim permission to be or to do whatever I feel like for no reason other
than that I feel like it
I claim self-love and nurturing
I claim the ability to protect myself from harm
I claim knowledge of what I want and don't want
I claim the ability to say no

I feel strongly that one should *not* view his or her body or illness as an enemy that must be fought and destroyed. This is just another form of resistance. It puts you in a negative relationship to *yourself* and I just can't see how any good could come from that.

A very important lesson I took from my illness is that how you define yourself has incredible power. People with chronic illness unconsciously alter their self-definitions over time. They may start out as people who feel strong and powerful or just ordinary, but gradually move toward feeling they are weak and helpless. I think it is okay, and even normal, to feel weak and helpless when you're sick. The trouble comes when you define your *self* as weak and helpless rather than your physical experience. You are still the strong and powerful person you were before the illness. This is so hard to remember. You certainly don't feel powerful! But, tell me, how can a weak and helpless person contribute anything towards their own healing?

It's tricky to make this leap in perception, but it is so powerful. I used the same technique when I quit smoking many years ago. After a few days with no cigarettes, the real struggle began. It was looking like I would head to the store for a pack, same as the last time and the time before that. Suddenly, I found myself looking at the situation differently. I clearly saw that my *addiction*, not my *self*, was the one running to the store. It was the *addiction* that couldn't quit. It was my addiction that didn't want to quit. *I* wanted to quit.

This amazing little revelation made all the difference to my success. It's like separating my ego from my intention. When the temptation to smoke got really strong, I would blame the temptation on the addiction and somehow this refusal to confuse the addiction with my self confirmed my conviction, and I was able to quit smoking for good. This same thing happens with illness. We start defining ourselves as our sickness and then everything is blurred and there is no *you* left around to help you to heal.

My mother was struggling with a batch of unfortunate physical circumstances and while I spoke with her on the telephone one evening, I could see that she had given away all her power. I was concerned she would be unable to get better, or to live a decent life with these circumstances since she defined herself as helpless. When I mentioned this to her, she was instantly grateful. It was immediately clear to her that she had forgotten herself, that she had mixed herself up with her illness, and that she would just sink into misery if she continued to do so.

For me, the second major healing shift was when I realized how much I had been allowing CFS to define me, how I had come to accept numerous limitations as my reality and how it was me who controlled all of this. I saw how I led with my illness. I was first someone with CFS. Sometimes I think I was *only* someone with CFS. When I began to challenge some of my beliefs, I saw how my expectations might be contributing to my experience.

And I want to talk about joy. This is so key to living with chronic illness that I can't stress it enough. When we are feeling lousy, it seems like there is no joy anywhere. And as we allow joy to recede further and further from our day-to-day lives, we sink lower and lower into our misery.

One beautiful summer when we had just moved to Seattle, I took to lounging around in a very comfortable hammock chair in my backyard. The differences in plants and birds from my home state of California kept me amused and engaged. I began to feel little bits of delight when a squirrel ran across my yard or a nuthatch stopped at the feeder. The rest was doing me good to be sure, but I noticed something else. I noticed tiny joy.

Now, joy, by it's very nature is huge, so even tiny joy is very big. These seconds that I felt stirrings of joy in my garden seemed to have a profound effect on me. I began noticing things that brought about this joy reaction. Trees, birds, music, sunsets, hugging my dog. I began to consciously add more and more of these small things to my every day and they gradually bumped out some rather dull things or even uncomfortable things that were taking up that time, just like eating vegetables makes you too full for junk food. The miracle of it was that I began to let go of the resentment that I had been carrying around towards my CFS. I could enjoy the fact that I wasn't working and could take a walk in the park in the middle of the week rather than pout that I was unable to work. The more I let joy in, the healthier I got; that is not exaggeration. Find your joy and then let it grow. Tiny joy is good. All joy is a powerful healer. Get some.

For all that we must let go of there are new things to embrace. This is no retreat—it is coming home to the pleasure of a cup of coffee after a good meal. It is the stillness of a resting bird. It is learning to really listen to the sounds around us. It is a gentle smile to keep to ourselves. It is pulling the curtain on your Mighty Oz, and clicking your heels together to get home to the truth. The journey is full of learning, learning, learning (some of it just felt like suffering, suffering, suffering!). Some of us need a bump on the head to take the walk into quiet time where we can behold the truth of our lives and our power.

Section 2

Specific Adaptive Strategies

Following are some strategies I have found to be helpful. The discovery of these strategies was an organic process for me. Only through hindsight could I see that I had, indeed, created my own treatment protocol. It could be bundled into steps and that didn't require that I exhaust myself chasing magic pills from medical professionals. I generally don't take much to formulaic wisdom, it just seems too tidy. On the other hand, it does help us to learn things in a way that doesn't require constantly referencing the source or teacher. In that spirit, I offer the following information in five "steps.' I recommend they be followed, at first, in the order they are listed. It can take months to move from one step to the next. Go at your own pace and be thorough.

I've tried not to be too redundant in this section, however, in some cases is has been necessary for me to make my point or to remind you of the way that I applied the step in my own experience. I also want this section to serve as a quick reference to the process without having to re-read Section One looking for something.

Remember that your recovery is a process of renewal and repair, reflection and self-compassion to which you commit every day. Once you have completed all the steps, you can go back and work on whichever area is called for. I find that this is an ongoing process and I have adapted my life to these steps, whether I am feeling completely well or not. Taking these steps on as a permanent lifestyle helps me to stay well enough to enjoy my life.

Real Rest

Rest is the first order of business when you have chronic fatigue syndrome. Your body is ill and your energy is needed on the inside for the time being. If you get the rest thing down you will find that you can get by on less of it eventually. But in the beginning it is crucial to lay low and let your body do the hard work of mending itself.

We know that people with CFS tend to have "non-restorative" sleep. That is, even with a good amount of sleep, we wake up feeling tired, as if we were just getting to bed after a full day—in fact sometimes feeling worse than when we went to bed the night before. It also means our bodies are not getting the recharging sleep is supposed to bring. I'm not sure the medical profession actually knows why this is, but it underscores the prominent role that rest must take in caring for and encouraging your body during this illness.

I have considered that CFS is the body-mind's way of forcing overworked or overwhelmed people to slow down. Recall that CFS occurs most commonly in overachiever types and often in people with a history of early truama who might have trouble feeling safe in the world. I know this rings a bit true in my own case. It is clear that, for me, a force such as this illness was the only way to get me to slow down! On the other hand I am also easily overwhelmed. Perhaps my over-achieving and fast pace had been a way to drown out the noise of my fear.

I have known many people with CFS who still insist they must do all of the housework, chauffeur friends and family around and pick up after their teen-aged children. Not so surprising to me that they have trouble getting better.

Rest doesn't come easy in our culture. One wants to avoid the label of "couch potato" or "lazy." At the same time, we praise people for taking a day off to lounge in the hammock. But it is conditional. There is an implied requirement that one must first work too hard to *earn* the rest period. It's not surprising to me that people with chronic illness have to struggle to allow themselves to rest. Many of us truly don't remember how. So let me spell it out some.

On the work front…if you are like many of us, you go to work sick. It is expected in the workplace culture, and that has created fear of being looked upon unfavorably by superiors if we do stay home with a cold. All of us have experienced co-workers hacking away with some horrible respiratory illness at the copy machine or in the cubical next door. I don't know how we got ourselves to this point but I find it rare to meet people who actually take the time their body needs to repair when they fall ill. A chronic illness will gradually force you to. It will shout louder and louder until you listen. So listen early and save yourself from feeling worse than you already do. Whatever you can. Recovery can be a full-time job in itself!

Work is a very tricky area because one's livelihood is at stake. In my experience, many of us underestimate what is possible for us financially. We are quick to say "But I *have* to work!" or to think that the CFS will go away in just another week or month. It can be very hard to expand the mind.

You may qualify for disability benefits from your employer or for Social Security Disability benefits from the U.S. government. Do some math and figure what you really can get by on. What is the bottom line? Perhaps you can get by on much less money working for a lower wage at a job that is less stressful in which you can be happier. Either way, rest is vital. Consider a leave of absence, reduced hours or job sharing. If you don't like your job, seriously explore quitting. Remember that things are never static. Just because you downshift your career efforts for now doesn't mean the change or break is forever.

You have to do your own work around this, but please take a good close look. It is such an important piece of the recovery process. Try writing out all of your fixed monthly expenses like rent and utilities. See what you might be able to alter. Can you do with fewer television channels? Can student loans be deferred? What about making minimum payments on your credit card for the time being or doing without internet access? Could you get rid of that second phone line or cell phone?

Another way we can get much-needed rest is by letting go of social, household and other commitments. Practice making tentative plans. Pace yourself. As I developed a pace that adapted to my CFS, I found that it was important for me to rest between tasks. I don't generally schedule more than one away-from-home thing in any day, even if they are hours apart. I rarely say I will absolutely be somewhere or do something so I can gauge my energy level at the time of the event. Of course, I place a priority on important occasions, but some of these I may miss and it can be a challenge to allow that to happen. Overachievers overbook themselves. Make whole blank days on your calendar a goal. If it's a work day, see about staying in that night. If I plan any activity for the better part of one day, I leave the next day blank so that I can be quiet and rest. Remember that you will be able to loosen up on these changes once you are better. It's just for now, for you.

Another challenge to doing less is the pressure we, and sometimes others, put on ourselves to be productive. I mention this earlier in this book. Treat yourself to a whole lot of compassion, love and understanding. Resting *is* doing. I have said that had I allowed myself this relatively simple thing, I might have recovered years earlier than I did. Years! Think of it.

Nap when you feel like it. I find it difficult to fall asleep in the daytime but if I really get to feeling sleepy I will lay down and rest. This is my form of napping. And it is a form of self love to hear the body ask for rest and to respond by stopping your activity. Why do we fight our own bodies so? It is so disrespectful. It creates a negative relationship between the mind and the body. What is that about? How does that make any sense? Is this what we want?

You've probably read a lot about meditation. This is another way to rest as long as you aren't a fretful meditator! Sitting quietly while watching the breath or repeating a mantra or pondering a tree benefits us by calming the mind along with the body. Studies have shown that it also reduces depression and blood pressure and can improve immune system function. Pay attention to your breathing. Shallow breathing from the chest can be a stress response. Inhaling and exhaling through alternate nostrils can be very soothing as it quiets the nervous system. There are various forms of nostril breathing. The one I like the best begins with long slow breaths in and out of the same nostril, repeating on the other side and ending with alternately breathing in one nostril—holding for a second—and breathing out the other using your fingers to close one side at a time.

Remember to say no when you need to. This is more of a problem for some of us than others. It is important for a very good reason. Have you ever observed a situation in which a person feels obligated to do something they really don't want to do? I have seen that the stronger the person feels that obligation and the more aversive the task, the more likely he or she is to come down with a sudden cold or flu just at the time of the dreaded event. It reminds me of the game of racing cars until someone chickens out—like in the James Dean movie, *Rebel Without A Cause.* As the event (or cliff) gets closer and your mind keeps telling you that you must go forward, the body pulls out at the last minute and says, "No way. I won't go." Don't force your body to pull that move. Say no when you mean no, and don't say yes unless you really mean it. If you feel you need permission to say no, spend some time exploring that. This life is precious. And it is short.

Learn to set limits. This is a neighbor to no. I always have a real hard time telling family and friends that I can't tolerate lengthy visits or phone calls. This alone is a big reason that people with CFS hang out with each other more than with their healthy friends. They don't need to explain and are usually keenly aware and thoughtful of each other's limitations. How does a healthy person relate to the exhaustion created just by keeping yourself alert enough to participate in a conversation? I remember so many times when I would tell people I was too tired to do something and they'd say, "That's alright. We don't have to do anything. We'll just sit around." How do you explain that just having a visitor in the room, no matter how beloved, is tiring and certainly not restful. It is the break from routine that exhausts, having to be present for something or struggling with a deep-seated need to please the other and ignore one's own needs.

If you have trouble sleeping, as many of us do, take some action. A lot of people take low doses of prescription medications, perhaps rotating different types to avoid becomming dependent. Some find the herb valerian or melatonin to be very helpful. A warm bath an hour before bedtime can help to make us sleepy. Moderate exercise earlier in the evening can help us fall into a good sleep. Just use caution and don't overdo. We are often quick to judge ourselves—not good enough, long enough, hard enough, fast enough—when exercising. Suspend the judgments and remember the goal is to love yourself enough to take care of yourself. Light exercise, including stretching, may help you sleep better. It's not marathon training. I do find that the less active I am during the day, the poorer the quality of my sleep. But with CFS, how active is too active and how inactive too inactive? You have to work with yourself and learn your own limits.

Detoxifying

Whether you've paid much attention to it or not, toxins are all around us in this day and age. We breath toxic substances in our air, drink them in our water, eat them in our foods in the form of pesticides or added chemicals. They are everywhere and so it is easy to overlook and underestimate their presence and impact.

It seems obvious enough to me that if your body is trying to get well, it isn't helped by dosing on chemicals of any kind. When your body encounters a foreigner—in my case, CFS—the immune system goes into action to get rid of the offender. The same thing happens when it encounters an environmental toxin. Where do you want your immune system to focus its attention? The goal should be less work for the immune system. You rest so it can do its job better. You don't want to add to its burden.

Below, I've listed a number of areas to investigate for toxic substances in your life. These are the more obvious ones. You may find more on your own but this will certainly get you started.

Household cleaners. There are lots of non-chemical cleaners available today in supermarkets and there are several good books with recipes for making your own out of common ingredients.

Carpets. Many people with CFS have multiple allergies and sensitivities. Carpets harbor dust mites, pet dander, molds and more. Throw rugs that can be shaken out and washed are preferable. Chemicals are often used in the backing and installation of wall-to-wall and other carpeting.

Water. Drink lots of water and make sure it's filtered or bottled. Cook with this water also. Wash your produce with it.

Food. Eat organic foods, especially grains, produce, and if you drink them—coffee and tea. Avoid junk foods and heavily processed, nutrient-challenged foods. Plants contain many complex biochemicals that have been found to protect and detoxify the body. These consist mostly of fruit, vegetables, unadulterated grains, green tea, beans, flax seed. Watch what you eat. I don't believe there is one diet for all bodies. Find what is right for you. Pay attention to the way eating certain foods make you feel. A lot of people have food allergies that can be detected through blood and stool tests. Avoid foods that cause an obvious reaction. Food allergies can be responsible for a wide range of symptoms including headache, rashes, joint pain, anxiety, fatigue, mood swings and many other unpleasant effects you wouldn't ordinarily think of attributing to your diet. Again, the idea is to let the immune system rest by taking away things that make it work overtime.

Linens. Use natural fabrics for your bedding. You can purchase special mattresses and pillows that are hypo-allergenic but all the ones I've ever seen are prohibitively expensive for many people. Change your bedding frequently. Wash in hot water with a few drops of eucalyptus oil, which kills dust mites and their eggs.

Bad habits. Avoid caffeine, sugar, alcohol, cigarettes (including second hand smoke), legal and illegal drugs of all kinds. Don't eat in restaurants that have smoking sections or, if you must, request a seat farthest from the smoking area.

Heavy metals. If your mouth is full of mercury amalgam fillings and you have the financial means and a knowledgeable dentist to do the work, you could have them carefully removed and replaced with non-toxic material that is readily available today. This topic is controversial, as the American Dental Association maintains that mercury fillings are benign. However, mercury is known to be a highly toxic substance and it is apparently indisputable that mercury vapors are released in the mouth when chewing. More and more dentists and scientists are supporting the removal of dental fillings that contain mercury. I do have a couple of friends that have had this work done and report significant decrease in pain and an increase in overall function. It is not a panacea. Just one of the many bits, and perhaps a fairly large bit at that, that you can do to support your health and immunity.

Candidiasis. Have your doctor check you out for lingering pathogens that might sabotage your recovery, like Candida Albicans, a naturally occurring yeast substance in the healthy flora of the digestive system. An overgrowth of this yeast, called Candidiasis, can be exposed with a stool sample. Naturopathic physicians are very familiar with this. Candida can grow out of control in the body, spurred by over-use of antibiotics, hormonal changes in women, the use of steroids or unhealthy eating habits and effect you in many ways, producing symptoms of fatigue, brain-fog, aches, digestive disturbances, headache and more. A significant number of people with CFS have been found to have candida overgrowth as a contributing factor to their illness. Many are completely recovered or nearly so by re-establishing a healthy gut. Treatment includes taking anti-fungal herbs or medications and a diet free of sugar, yeast, known food allergens and simple car-bohydrates. You may need to see a naturopath (N.D.) for diagnosis and treat-ment, as some M.D.'s are skeptical or unaware of the role candida can play.

Body care. Don't wear perfume or use scented body products. Stay away from magazines that contain perfume strips. I've noticed that I react to the inks in cer-tain magazines, especially some of the art magazines with heavy graphics. Use simple, natural soaps and shampoos with few ingredients. Don't polish your fin-gernails; both the polish and the remover are toxic and many of their ingredients are known carcinogens. Non-toxic alternatives may be availble in your area.

Plastic. Plastic products do what is called "outgassing." I don't claim to under-stand this, but prefer glass, wood, plain paper or natural wicker over plastic con-tainers in my home.

Fumes. Avoid car and bus fumes. If I am out for a walk, I use secondary streets so that I am not breathing the exhaust from traffic on the busier roads. Consider where you live. If there is a lot of traffic, don't keep doors and windows open that face the busy street. Open the opposite end of the house for fresh air.

Your environment. Notice toxins where you live, walk, work and in your car. Make over all of the environments where you spend a significant amount of your time. Avoid places where a lot of chemicals are used such as home remodels and beauty salons. I don't even walk down the cleanser aisle in supermarkets. I figure if I can smell too much chemical smell, I don't want to get close to it.

Air. Invest in an air purifier with a hepa filter. Keep heater and other vents cleaned.

Buildings. Avoid freshly painted or carpeted rooms.

Your Mouth. Practice good dental hygiene to keep bacteria down—another potential distraction for the immune system.

Joy

So once you are resting and have reduced the distractions from your body's work of getting well from CFS, take some time to focus your attention on the very valuable idea of joy.

Joy has tremendous healing potential. Read *Anatomy of An Illness*; Norman Cousins' work on humor and wellness. Recall the studies that have shown that smiling has a positive impact on mood, regardless of whether or not the smile was genuine. Yet another study demonstrated that when people were shown a beautiful view, there was a chemical reaction in the body that lifted the spirits. Lifted spirits are good for you. With joy, muscles relax and thus, function better and feel less painful. The immune system is given a boost. The breath gets deeper, setting off a chain of beneficial physical and psychological events.

Where is the joy in your life? It seems a bit of a paradox and you might have trouble feeling joyful in your condition, but look at it as a prescription for wellness and understand that joy is a powerful force, so a little goes a long way.

Joy doesn't require much from you. It's a matter of recognizing what brings you joy and then filling your life with as much of it as you can. In my life, most joy is free. I get it from watching my pets, listening to music, watching the sun set or looking at a beautiful tree. When you are in pain, try noticing the parts of your body that aren't hurting or that are engaged in other things like feeling a breeze on your skin or the weight and warmth where your cat lays against you. Extend your noticing to the beautiful green of a houseplant or the dappled sunlight coming in through the blinds. See the clouds moving across the sky, the bird at the feeder. Notice the comfort of your chair. In exercising the noticing of all things, we find that there are spaces where life is good. There is this good and there is this tiredness. We may then notice that the tiredness or the pain is all we have been tending to—it has been so loud. With practice, the joy can be heard above the din of the discomfort.

For some reason, I have found that people have trouble with this concept. When they are feeling miserable, joy sounds like too much work. But joy can be simple and can bring great benefit. If all you can do is sit in a chair or lay on a couch, why not have someone hang a birdfeeder out the window so you can watch the songbirds come to treat. If blue is your favorite color, why aren't you wearing blue pajamas? If you love the feel of sateen sheets, have them on your bed. If you've got a moment of energy, why waste it doing the dishes? Ask what part of you—or habit in you—is putting household chores above all else. Take a walk in a lovely park instead. Or around your house if that is all the energy you have. And when you're walking, or just sitting outside, notice nature. Immerse yourself in the smells and colors of the season. Let yourself feel the gratitude for the beauty of a magnificent tree. Connect.

I encourage you to make a list, writing down as many things as you can think of that give you joy. Really work at this list. Get into some details. What colors do you love? Flavors? Smells? When you are done—and I hope you have many pages and add to it whenever you're inspired—examine your list and consider how many of these joys you have in your life right now. How do you want to spend your time?

Sadly, this is an eye-opening exercise for many of us. We see that joy has not been much of a priority. At the same time, it encourages us to see how joy can be found in the very simplest of things. Make a commitment to bringing as many of the things on your list as you possibly can into your life.

To help get you started, here's a partial list of my own:

- Pink puppy bellies

- Singing Beatles songs

- Holding babies

- Colorful, magnificent flowers

- Reading poetry

- Fresh air

- Dancing of any kind

- Hugging

- Talking with good friends

- Art books

- Birdwatching

- The feel of warm sun on bare skin

- Ice cream

- Fresh-baked cookies

- The smell of lilacs

- Blooming dogwood trees

- Sparkly glass beads

- Walking on the beach; sand in bare feet

- Reading under a tree

- Watching it snow

- The sound of ocean waves

- Laying in grass

- Fat socks

- Candles in the winter

- The sound of Tibetan singing bowls

- Writing in a journal

- Making a collage out of magazine pictures

- Watching clouds move across the sky

- The sound of rain on the roof

- Sitting quietly on the deck

- Eating out

- Pudding

- Hot bubble baths

- fleece throws in sage green

Self-Exploration

o o o o o o o o o o o o o o o o o o o o o o o o o o o o o o o o o

*"There is nothing that is not path. Daily practice, no cramming;
Consistency, not crisis."*

—*Mark Ian Barasch, The Healing Path*

We, as patients, don't always see is the role we play in our own healing. Doctors and their treatments are external. *We* are responsible for our interior. Let's face it, there is no answer good enough if it's not a quick cure. We see the doctor's role as prescribing and our role as taking the presecription and that's that. We have forgotten the part where we take care of ourselves. Our culture continuously reminds us that we are expected to cover up our symptoms with medicine and then continue through our daily to-do lists as if nothing is changed.

So now it's time to do some exploring. This step asks that you go inside and reach for any possible part that your mind is playing in your illness. It's a tough one to tackle. Many people are immediately put off by any suggestion that they are contributing to their own situation. Try to look at it instead as taking back some power. I do believe we have control over *some* of our situation and that we can gain not only better health, but some relief from our sense of powerlessness if we do this work. It is not shameful to admit we have a subconscious mind that often works in ways of which we are largely unaware.

I am not offended by the notion of my CFS as a teacher. Teachers are all around us. Anyone or anything can be a teacher. Some people have profound experiences swimming with dolphins. Their lives may be changed after a single encounter. The dolphin has been their teacher in that moment. Others are impacted by books, parents, the I Ching, movies, lovers, insects, strangers. Teachers are everywhere in our lives and in every moment. Our intention, openness and ability to listen is what sets the learning in motion. The teachers are always there whether we are tuned to them or not.

The lessons I have learned—and continue to learn—from my illness are many. The first and most obvious was to slow down. My life became measurably richer when I released myself from the chains and sense of urgency to get things done so common in our culture. It was difficult at first, as I struggled with my body, unwilling and unable to accept inactivity, but gradually I woke up to see the value of stillness.

Remember when "voluntary simplicity" was a new and popular concept? I had taken to calling my own situation "involuntary simplicity," but you know, I have tried to hang onto that simplicity as my health improved. So what began as involuntary is now whole-heartedly voluntary.

The simpler and less complicated I make my life, the more restful my spirit, the more time to appreciate everything around me, the less likely I am to make myself sick with stress and overwork. I live for the moments walking on the beach, resting on my deck under the magnificent cedar trees in my yard, or finding myself baking cookies without having had any plans to do so. Keeping things simple allows room for these things. It creates space for us to manifest something more in our lives—preferably something that doesn't feel busy!

During this phase of exploration, begin asking yourself some tough questions. Be open with yourself and approach this time with honesty and compassion. Give yourself permission to see into your behavior without judgment. There is nothing to be ashamed of. Nothing to hide from yourself. No punishment. Love yourself enough to do the work.

I've included some questions here that may help to get you started. You may decide that many or all of them don't apply to your situation. The benefit is in the exploration. If you find something that rings true for you, go with that. I believe that sometimes we may create or at least perpetuate ill health on a subconscious level when we don't want to face, or don't have the courage to face, something in our lives.

I also realize that I am blessed to have reached the level of recovery that I have. I know that some people with CFS are unable to get out of bed for years at a time. I hope that all can accept these questions in the spirit they are intended. It is worth the satisfaction of resolving anything that might be holding us back or creating undo stress in our lives.

Do you feel overwhelmed by your life? Too many commitments or responsibilities? Too many people counting on you? Not enough time in the day? Are you sometimes frightened by the amount of responsibility you carry? Do you ever wonder how you manage to pull it off? Do you ask for help when you need it? Do you feel that if you took time away from your responsibilities at home or work that things would fall apart? Could your illness be your body's way of forcing you to back off? Or could being sick be perhaps the only way you would give yourself permission to take a real break or initiate a big change?

Do you frequently find it difficult to say no when someone asks for a favor or when you receive an invitation to a party or family function? Does a loved one at home or a colleague at work rely on you heavily? Do you live to please others? Are people dropping by to visit or calling to talk on the phone when you need to rest, but you don't know how to ask them to stop? Do you let your boss or your family know when they are piling too much work on your desk? Or do you silently fume and push on through? Is it easier for you to tell people no because you are sick than just to say no without offering any explanation? Why do you think that is?

Do you find inactivity deplorable? Are you *only* okay if you're being productive? Are you easily upset by laziness in others? Do you judge others by their productivity or accomplishments? What would it mean if you learned that you, in fact, are lazy yourself? Could you ever give yourself permission to make room for some laziness in your life? Could illness be the only acceptable excuse for inactivity in your mind? What if the body needs to slow down? Is that okay? What if the absolute truth is that you want to be irresponsible and lazy lazy lazy? Could you not be harsh with yourself and figure out an acceptable way to bring less responsibility and more down-time into your life? Could you allow someone else to do that?

Could you be afraid of life? Are you inclined to withdraw? Does a part of you want to disappear from all of your commitments and/or the judgement of others? I used to think that perhaps I was being exhausted by the amount of courage I needed to screw up just to be in the world. Did something scary happen that made you afraid to go outside and interact with people? Did someone or something hurt you very badly? Is a part of you avoiding life like a child's hand might avoid a hot stove? Are you scared? Does being sick get you out of having to go "out there" and place yourself in threatening situations? Could you or do you have a history of emotional or physical abuse? Social phobias? Agoraphobia? Could they somehow be connected to the CFS? The role of repressed emotions cannot be understated. Get help if you need it.

Did your mother or other caregiver fuss over you when you were sick as a child? Shame you for not doing enough? Does anyone today? Do you tell everyone your latest symptoms without having been asked? When you meet someone new, do you tell them you are sick before a second meeting? When do you tell them? Do you hide it? Do you have a strong support system? Are you touched enough?

Think of other questions to explore on your own. You may have a clue already where to go with it. If you stumble on something, take the appropriate action. Learn to speak your mind or to allow some self-pampering. Take the time and love yourself enough.

Consider committing yourself to lifestyle changes that are permanent. It's kind of like when people pray and make promises to do (or not do!) certain things if their prayers are answered. If you get well, will you go back to your old ways? What would you change? How can you convince your body-mind that you will take care of it in the future? That you don't need it to force the issue by making or keeping you sick, but that you will make an honest commitment to restore and maintain balance in your life once you are well.

Minding Our Perceptions

*"If there is anything like a law of consciousness, it is this: Whatever
we focus our attention on expands in our lives."*

—Laurence G. Boldt, The Tao of Abundance

*"We are in relationship with our expectations and not with life itself.
Which brings up the idea that we may become as wounded by the
way in which we see an illness as by the illness itself."*

—Rachel Naomi Remen, Kitchen Table Wisdom

Now you are ready for the final step. It may be the most important step of
all—but not without completing the other steps first. You can continue to work
the previous steps after your work with this last one, but do so because they're in
your best interest, not because you are sick.

While it was necessary to spend a lot of time adjusting to meeting the needs
you have had as a sick person, now the challenge is to erase all such thoughts. The
quote above says it well. The more time you spend thinking and talking and act-
ing about your illness the more you become swallowed up by it.

Remember how I mentioned that I came to feel like I ate, breathed, talked and
slept sickness. Every moment I seemed to be evaluating the CFS. If I was tired I
blamed the it on the illness. Same thing if I couldn't conjure up a word or find
my car keys. This may have served me at one time but I could see that it had hold
of me in an unhealthy way. I was smart to wonder if I could be perpetuating my
illness by focusing so much attention on it and identifying so strongly with it.
Just as I had once asked, "Who would I be without my job?" now I had to ask,
"Who am I without my illness?."

It seemed like at that time I was being called back to the drawing board. I had
dug myself right into a hole! Now I had all these beliefs about my health that,
well, weren't healthy! I had given all of my power away. I realized that I felt afraid

to stray from the routine and rituals I had created to get well. Could it be that these very things were now keeping me sick?

Almost the instant I got this idea in my head I felt much healthier. That was the point when I went back to work and I have been working ever since—that was in 1996! I continue to work my steps, but they have become natural for me. I believe they support my continued good health. But I must be careful not to believe so hard that I am afraid to step outside the lines. That is where the trouble lies.

When I realized that I didn't want to identify so closely with my illness, I gave all of my CFS books to the local support group. I had a least a dozen of them. I stopped subscribing to journals and chronicles on CFS. In fact, I took a break from all health-related meanderings, including all magazines and television shows. I stopped relating the current state of my health in letters and conversations. I felt a real need for a time-out. Too much focus is understandable because we want to get well and because the symptoms can be so loud. But there is a point where it is self-defeating, keeping us stuck because that is where our energy and attention is going.

It's not just that you are sick, it's what you attach to being sick that can complicate things. At the moment in any day when you have the thought, "I feel so lousy and sick," notice the thoughts that immediately follow. I'll bet they aren't positive. Do they tell you anything about how you view yourself and your illness? How long do you continue with these internal, self-bashing follow-up thoughts? The original thought was that you felt sick. What's all this other stuff? Is it helping you or hurting you? Does it belong there? What would happen if you just sit with the original thought and don't add any commentary? Can you see how we pile on expectations and judgements that only hurt us more?

In earlier times in some cultures women removed themselves to specially designated quarters during their menstrual periods. They dropped their usual chores and responsibilities for several days. They didn't fret over this interruption or about what wasn't getting done, but just relaxed and enjoyed the forced quieting of their ordinary lives. They were able to luxuriate in this time, taking advantage of the opportunity to appreciate the company of other women. Wouldn't it be nice if we could view our own relapses so casually. No fear. No worries. Nothing more important to do than stop and care for ourselves.

When I went back to work, I decided I didn't want to spend more than thirty hours a week on the job. I avoided playing the, "because I have CFS" card although I admit I did use it when an employer wanted to expand my hours to forty a week. I simply noticed that when I worked forty hour weeks there was no time left to spend with joy and rest, my two new lovely companions. I present the thirty hours as a preference. Not a have-to-or-I'll-be-sick. Can you allow a preference priority-status in your life? I hope so.

I know this might sound crazy or hard to understand. I hope I can communicate it so that you can get something out of it, because I feel it is such an important step. Get rid of all thoughts of CFS. Lose it all. Live your life. Say no when you have to. Nap when you want to. Forget a word once in awhile and don't make it mean anything. Cease the constant measuring of symptoms and their severity. Get up early once in a while and don't fret over how tired you might (or might not!) feel that day. Learn to honor your preferences in life without judgement—even if you find that you prefer to sleep in until 11:00 every morning—and without needing something to blame it on (like CFS.) Stop stressing over how long you'll be sick or if you'll get worse. Just give it all up. Just let whatever is be. Resist the call to judge it or label it.

The tendency to want to assign a cause or reason or blame for every symptom is our way of trying to control the illness, but it can ultimately sabotage our ability to regain functioning because a great deal of the time, the cause we assign is false.

The other day I suddenly got a post nasal drip. I wondered what it was I had done to cause it. Hmmmm. My husband had swept the floors and I could be sensitive to dust or to the dander from my two dogs. He had also raked the yard and it's fall so it likely had stirred up some mold. Was it my new shampoo? The exhaust from my neighbors dryer vent? The wood burning in the fireplace? Any of these could be the culprit and the fact is: I may never know.

So go easy on yourself and forget trying to figure it all out. Let go of all of it and just be with what is in this moment. Don't expect marathons for now. Don't expect anything in particular. Read. Walk gently. Pull up a chair overlooking a lake or the ocean. Set limits with friends (short visits!). Work part time or from home if you want. Fill your life with joyful things that are passive. Begin by creating a life for yourself that you can do sick, so that your limitations aren't always in your face. Be gentle with yourself. Breathe deeply. Live deeply. It doesn't have to be noisy or fast to be real living.

Recommended Reading

The Alchemy of Illness, Kat Duff

Anatomy of An Illness, Norman Cousins

Healing Back Pain, John Sarno

The Highly Sensitive Person, Elaine N. Aron

Home Safe Home, Debra Lynn Dadd

Running on Empty, Katrina H. Berne

Sounds of Healing, Mitchell Gaynor

Still Here, Ram Dass

Transforming Trauma: EMDR, Laurel Parnell

The Woman's Comfort Book, Jennifer Louden

The Yeast Connection, William Crook

Anything by SARK

Kitchen Table Wisdom, Rachel Naomi Remen

My Grandfather's Blessing, Rachel Naomi Remen

0-595-32609-9